PEDIATRIC COLLECTIONS
Dermatology Cases

EDITED BY:

Miriam Weinstein, BSc, BScN, MD, FRCPC (Paediatrics), FRCPC (Dermatology)
Pediatrics in Review Editorial Board
Member, Section of Dermatology, AAP
Associate Professor, University of Toronto
Paediatric Dermatologist, The Hospital for Sick Children
Toronto, Ontario, Canada

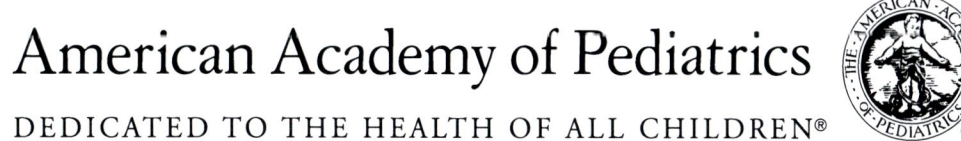

American Academy of Pediatrics
DEDICATED TO THE HEALTH OF ALL CHILDREN®

Published by the American Academy of Pediatrics
345 Park Blvd.
Itasca, IL 60143

The American Academy of Pediatrics is not responsible for the content of the resources mentioned in this publication. Web site addresses are as current as possible but may change at any time. Products are mentioned for information purposes only. Inclusion in this publication does not imply endorsement by the American Academy of Pediatrics.

APC040

Print ISBN: 978-1-61002-775-5
eBook ISBN: 978-1-61002-776-2

PEDIATRIC COLLECTIONS
Dermatology Cases

Table of Contents

Dermatology Cases: Case Reports from *Pediatrics in Review*

About AAP Pediatric Collections

Pediatric Collections is a series of selected pediatric articles that highlight different facets of information across various AAP publications, including AAP Journals, AAP News, Blog Articles, and eBooks. Each series of collections focuses on specific topics in the field of pediatrics so that you can keep up with best practices and make an informed response to public health matters, trending news, and current events. Each collection includes previously published content focusing on specific topics and articles selected by AAP editors.

Visit http://collections.aap.org to view current online collections.

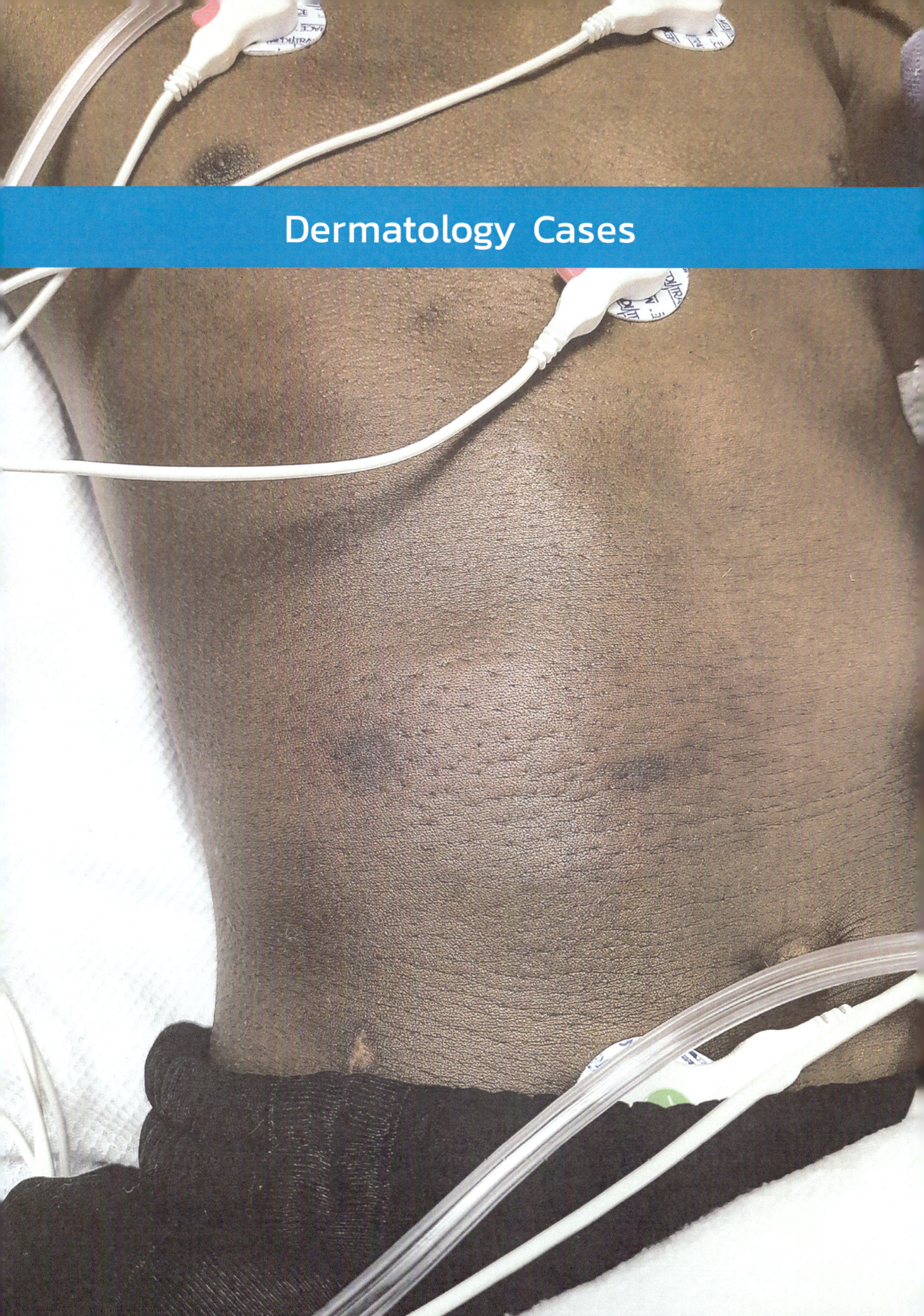

Dermatology Cases

Dermatology Cases
Collection Introduction

Miriam Weinstein, BSc, BScN, MD, FRCPC (Paediatrics), FRCPC (Dermatology)
Pediatrics in Review Editorial Board
Member, Section of Dermatology, AAP
Associate Professor, University of Toronto
Paediatric Dermatologist, The Hospital for Sick Children
Toronto, Ontario, Canada

"Can you have a quick look at this picture?" This is a question I'm asked almost daily, before being shown images of lesions, rashes, and various skin findings. "Of course I can have a quick *look*!" is my typical response before promptly adding, "however, I *think* slowly!" My quick look at the photo is always followed by asking many questions—about the patient's history, other cutaneous features, and findings on the physical exam. This highlights the importance of the clinical reasoning and critical thinking that underlie the diagnostic process. Even when I think I know what the issue might be upon first look, I want to put the morphologic findings into context.

The ability in dermatology to literally see and touch the disease directly offers great diagnostic information but has the potential to lead us astray. The art of visual literacy involves looking at the morphology but interpreting what is seen in the context of the patient's history, the cutaneous exam, and the general physical exam. The process can range from rapid pattern recognition to complex detective work. Even in cases where a "spot" diagnosis is possible, considering those other sources of information allows one to confirm the first impression. For example, I may see a couple of small, well-demarcated, red plaques with a thick silvery scale on the lower arms of a patient and rapidly make a diagnosis of psoriasis. However, a full exam might show the rest of the lesions are tiny, most prominent on the trunk, and the history might reveal a recent strep throat infection. The diagnosis of guttate psoriasis, secondary to group A streptococcal infection—the correct diagnosis in this scenario—is related to psoriasis, but unique in presentation and management and needs to be distinguished from classic plaque psoriasis.

The recent dermatology case reports from *Pediatrics in Review* presented in this collection were chosen to highlight several different ways of thinking about dermatologic conditions in children. The articles are randomly assorted and not specifically grouped to reflect these different perspectives and, of course, some case presentations will fit more than one category! There are a few articles that present patients with uncommon variants of relatively common pediatric skin conditions. This provides a reminder that even classic conditions can have varied presentations that can be challenging to diagnose.

A second group of articles present findings that on initial presentation can be alarming; for example, patients with certain genital lesions or acute pigmented lesions. These articles will provide context and examples to help the reader remain alert to concerning conditions or situations and to also appreciate other less-concerning causes for similar findings.

There are several cases presenting congenital or acquired "lumps and bumps" that are moderately common in a pediatric dermatology practice and are a common source of referrals from primary care and consulting pediatric practitioners. Learning more about these conditions may enable readers to recognize them, help distinguish them from mimickers, and be aware of when the cutaneous findings may be a sign of associated systemic features.

There are several reports of patients with rare rashes that can have a significant risk for systemic morbidity. Being alert to the ways in which these conditions present will prepare the practitioner to consider these entities when assessing patients with similar presentations. While the focus of this collection is on morphology, relevant history, and the diagnostic process, we have many innovative treatments that we use in dermatology, and thus one article focuses on an innovative treatment.

The authors of these patient presentations have presented important, informative, and interesting cases from which I learned a great deal. I invite you to read the collection! My hope is that this collection of cases will increase your knowledge of skin diseases in children, encourage you to appreciate how morphology of skin disease can provide a wealth of diagnostic clues, reinforce information you already know, and challenge you to think about the diverse presentations of dermatologic presentations.

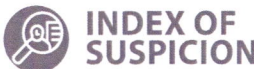

INDEX OF SUSPICION

Facial Lesions and Rash in a 2-month-old Boy

Alexandra Curry, DO,* Anoop Khalsa, MD,* David Yi, DO*

*Department of Pediatrics, University of California San Francisco–Fresno, Fresno, CA

PRESENTATION

A 2-month-old former term boy with no known medical conditions presented with a 1-month history of persistent scabbed lesions on his face and scalp and 2 weeks of a worsening rash on his arms, legs, palms, and soles. According to the mother, the scalp lesion was present at birth, and she continues to peel the scab during bathing. There was no scalp probe, vacuum, or forceps used at delivery. The facial lesions were initially ulcerative and then developed scabs but did not heal completely. The rash began on the extremities and spread proximally. He has no other symptoms. His sister was recently diagnosed as having scabies and is currently being treated. Per mom, there has not been any recent travel, hiking or camping, animal exposures, tick bites, or ingestions other than his regular formula.

Two weeks before delivery, his mother developed a painful vesicular vaginal lesion without associated regional lymphadenopathy after unprotected intercourse with a new partner. She received no testing of her lesion but was prescribed empirical acyclovir during the last 2 weeks of pregnancy because she was positive for herpes simplex virus (HSV) type 2 IgG antibody. The lesion was reportedly still present but was healing the day of delivery, when mom had a precipitous vaginal delivery. Mom had no other pertinent medical history. Her prenatal laboratory test results were negative for hepatitis B, human immunodeficiency virus, and group B streptococcus. She also had 3 negative fluorescent treponemal antibody absorption (FTA-Abs) test results at 31, 35, and 38 weeks' gestation, the last test being the day of delivery. At birth, the patient's examination findings were normal except for a round, 2-cm, raised lesion on his scalp. HSV surface cultures and HSV blood polymerase chain reaction were negative at that time.

On presentation to the emergency department he is afebrile and his other vital signs are within normal limits, with weight at 5,578 g (36th percentile) and height at 23.8 in (60.5 cm) (69th percentile), on track with his birth percentiles. On physical examination there is a diffuse, papulosquamous, blanchable, erythematous, targetoid, well-circumscribed, partially crusted rash that includes the palms, soles, and scalp, without mucosal involvement (Figs 1–3). He has several soft, palpable cervical lymph nodes less than 1 cm each, and the liver is palpable 2 cm below the subcostal margin.

Laboratory evaluation shows a white blood cell count of 10,700/μL (10.7×10^9/L), a hemoglobin level of 7.9 g/dL (79 g/L) with a mean corpuscular volume of 86.7 fL (86.7 μm^3), and a platelet count of 150×10^3/μL (150×10^9/L). The differential count is 63% lymphocytes and 22% neutrophils, 1% bands, 8% monocytes, 5% eosinophils, and 1% basophils. The C-reactive protein level is 10.75 mg/dL (107.5 mg/L)

AUTHOR DISCLOSURE: Drs Curry, Khalsa, and Yi have disclosed no financial relationships relevant to this article. This commentary does not contain a discussion of an unapproved/investigative use of a commercial product/device.

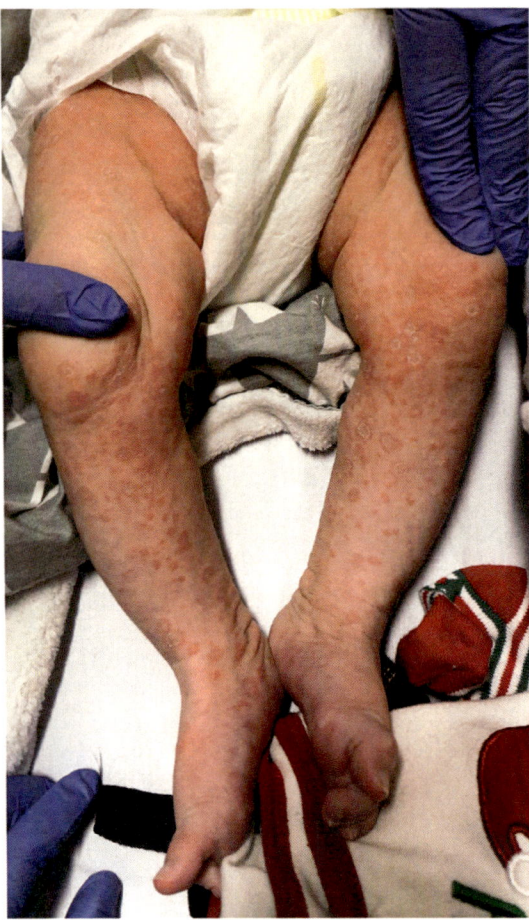

Figure 1. Healing scalp chancre over the right parietal bone.

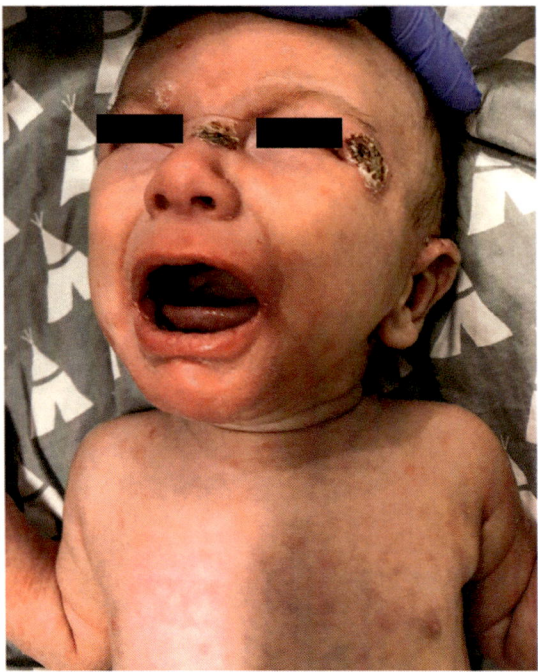

Figure 2. Scabbed facial chancre over the bridge of the nose and lateral to the left eye.

(reference range, 0–1.5 mg/dL [0–15.0 mg/L]). The procalcitonin level is 315 ng/dL (3.15 μg/L) (reference range, 0–30 ng/dL [0.3 μg/L]). His metabolic panel is within the reference range, including normal hepatic enzyme levels. COVID-19 polymerase chain reaction is negative. No imaging is performed. Pending laboratory results from his outside pediatrician and our facility ultimately help reveal the diagnosis.

DISCUSSION

Differential Diagnosis

The differential diagnosis includes rheumatologic, allergic, and infectious causes. Neonatal lupus erythematosus and psoriasis were considered but were less likely given a negative family history and the wide distribution and appearance of the rash. The skin targetoid lesions on the trunk and extremities were similar to a hypersensitivity response such as erythema multiforme, which could have been secondary to potential HSV infection. However, the crusted facial lesions were inconsistent with erythema multiforme, and his previous

postnatal HSV evaluation at birth was negative. Coxsackievirus, rickettsia, bacterial endocarditis, toxic shock syndrome, measles, and meningococcemia are potential organisms that could cause a rash on the palms, but the patient did not

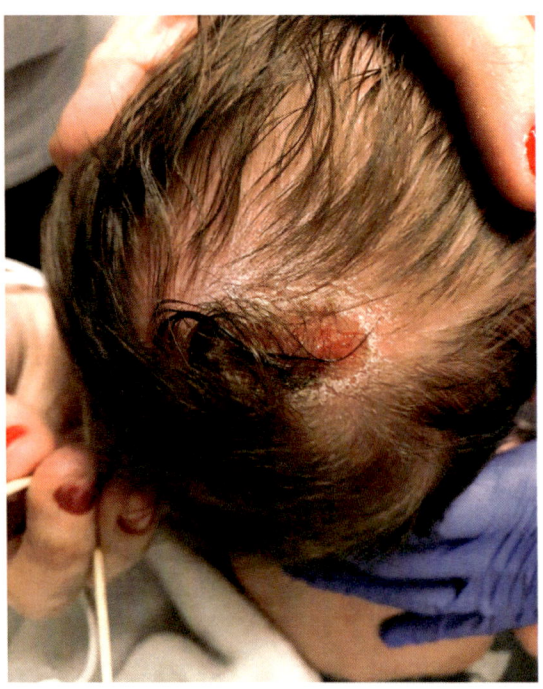

Figure 3. Generalized rash on the legs and soles.

have a fever, mucosal involvement, or other systemic symptoms that are seen with these infections. Given his sister's recent infection, we considered scabies; however, it is usually a pruritic rash with 3- to 5-mm papules often in the presence of pustules, unlike our patient's more confluent, targetoid rash. Maternal syphilis testing was negative, and her genital lesion was painful, which is more consistent with an HSV lesion. However, congenital syphilis was considered because the facial lesions exhibited a chancrelike appearance, and his painless maculopapular rash involving the palms and soles resembled a syphilitic infection, especially in the setting of his lymphadenopathy, anemia, and hepatomegaly. In addition, negative syphilis test results are possible, especially if testing is performed early in the disease process. The mom's new sexual encounter was approximately 2 weeks before delivery, and the FTA-Abs treponemal assay can take 3 to 4 weeks to become positive in primary syphilis. (1)(2)

Actual Diagnosis/Clinical Course and Management
On hospital day 2, the patient's rapid plasma reagin (RPR) titer was reactive at 1:256. Based on the laboratory and examination findings in the setting of a positive RPR, our patient was diagnosed as having early congenital syphilis. Of note, during our patient's admission, his mom tested positive for syphilis with an RPR of 1:128, therefore confirming that the infant was exposed to untreated maternal syphilis. He was not tested for syphilis at birth secondary to negative maternal testing because she was too early in her infection for the assays to accurately detect infection. A lumbar puncture was completed, and he was started on penicillin treatment. He was also treated empirically with acyclovir for HSV until the HSV blood culture, cerebrospinal fluid (CSF), and mucosal cultures were finalized as negative.

Two hours after the first dose of intravenous penicillin G, he became tachycardic, hypertensive, and febrile, with increased fussiness. A Jarisch-Herxheimer reaction was suspected. The patient was given 1 dose of acetaminophen, and he improved. There were no further reactions with subsequent penicillin G doses. The plain radiograph bone survey showed periostitis consistent with congenital syphilis; however, his remaining evaluation was largely negative. He had a nonreactive CSF-VDRL test result. Given the lack of pleocytosis or increased protein in the CSF, we had a low suspicion for neurosyphilis and, therefore, did not obtain a brain magnetic resonance image. (3)(5) The ophthalmologic examination findings and auditory brainstem response were normal. He completed a 10-day course of penicillin G. (6) He was discharged with scheduled follow-up. He missed his 3-month appointment, but testing 6 and 9 months after

treatment showed significant improvement; however, he continues to be seropositive, with an RPR at 1:2. He will follow up next at 12 months.

The Condition
Treponema pallidum is the spirochete that causes congenital syphilis. The incidence in the United States has continued to increase since 2013 and is currently 125 to 180 cases per 100,000 live births, highest among non-Hispanic American Indian or Alaskan Native, Pacific Islander, and Black or African American populations. (7)(8) In 2020, preliminary data show more than 2,000 cases of congenital syphilis, including 139 stillbirths or infant deaths. (7) In 2019, 50% of counties in the United States reported at least 1 case of syphilis (all stages) among women of reproductive age (15–44 years), which serves as an important reminder that congenital syphilis can be seen almost anywhere. (7)(8) Globally, congenital syphilis is a leading cause of preventable stillbirth, highlighting the importance of prenatal screening. (9)(10)

Syphilis is transmitted through the placenta or contact with infectious lesions during birth. Untreated syphilis during pregnancy has a rate of perinatal transmission of 60% to 100%. (3)(4)(5)(11) This rate is increased during the second half of pregnancy and is higher in mothers with primary or secondary syphilis. (12) Fetal or perinatal death occurs in 40% of infants born to infected and untreated moms. (3)(11) Patients may present as severe as hydrops fetalis and stillbirth, or they may be asymptomatic at birth and only develop signs and symptoms weeks to months later.

Because spirochetes widely disseminate, nearly all organ systems can be infected. Early findings (within the first 2 years after birth) include maculopapular erythematous rash involving copper red spots on the palms and soles; skin peeling; persistent copious rhinitis (snuffles); diffuse lymphadenopathy; pneumonitis; jaundice; hepatosplenomegaly; and pseudoparalysis of Parrot caused by painful osteochondritis or periostitis, which manifests as decreased movement of the extremities, mainly the upper limbs. Laboratory evaluation at birth or within the first 4 to 8 weeks of age most commonly reveals Coombs-negative hemolytic anemia, thrombocytopenia associated with platelet trapping in an enlarged spleen, and elevated liver enzyme levels secondary to bile stasis or fibrosis. (3)(6)

Late manifestations (after 2 years but within the first 2 decades) can be prevented by treatment of early infection. These manifestations include frontal bossing, keratitis, Hutchinson teeth, saddle nose, saber shins, gummas, and juvenile paresis, which occurs during adolescence and manifests as behavior changes, focal seizures, and loss of intellectual function. (3)(6)

Laboratory Diagnosis

There are 2 types of tests used to diagnose syphilis: nontreponemal and specific treponemal antibody tests. There are 2 algorithms used to determine management. (6) The classic or traditional pathway first uses a nontreponemal assay (eg, RPR and VDRL, which measure host antibodies made in response to phosphatidylcholine taken up from mammalian tissue by *T pallidum* during an active infection) and if positive is confirmed with a treponemal test (eg, manual FTA-Abs and *T pallidum* particle agglutination assay or automated enzyme immunoassay and chemiluminescence immunoassay, which measure antibodies to *T pallidum*). It takes 4 to 6 weeks after the initial infection for an RPR test to become reactive. Because the RPR is a marker of active infection, it may be negative in the setting of latent or late syphilis. The reverse algorithm, more often used now especially in endemic areas, performs a treponemal assay first, and should that be positive, is followed by a nontreponemal test. Treponemal antibodies appear earlier than nontreponemal antibodies, allowing for earlier detection of syphilis with the reverse algorithm. (1)(2)(3) Even still, it takes 3 to 4 weeks for the treponemal assays to be reactive in the setting of an infection, and in some literature, FTA-Abs testing was found to be less sensitive than other treponemal assays for primary syphilis (Table). (10)(13)(14) To this end, patients in high-risk areas with a history of a sexual encounter with a new partner late in pregnancy may need follow-up testing for syphilis because initial testing could have been before the ability of the assay to detect antibodies. In addition, symptomatic patients should receive both treponemal and nontreponemal testing. The FTA-Abs test involves the addition of fluorescein isothiocyanate–labeled anti–human globulin antibody to a patient's serum for the detection of anti–*T pallidum* antibody. The degree of fluorescence is then manually read based on the degree of fluorescence and is graded +1 to +4. False-negatives within the period of reactivity are rare and difficult to quantify but are due to either a human failure to quantify fluorescence on the slide or a decreased specificity of the fluorescein isothiocyanate–labeled anti–human globulin antibodies. (2)

Of note, qualitative treponemal tests should not be used in the diagnosis or treatment of infants because passive transplacental transfer of IgG maternal antibodies may persist until 15 months. (6)(15) Therefore, 1 of the diagnostic criteria for congenital syphilis is that the infant's nontreponemal titer (eg, RPR) is at least 4-fold greater than the mother's titer at birth, indicating fetal antibody synthesis. It is important to consider the history of maternal treatment and her nontreponemal titer response while planning the infant evaluation and management. The following evaluation is warranted when congenital syphilis is suspected: CSF-VDRL test, cell count and protein level; complete blood cell count with differential count; and other tests as clinically indicated, including liver function tests, human immunodeficiency virus testing, long-bone and chest radiographs, abdominal ultrasonography, neuroimaging, and ophthalmologic and auditory brainstem examinations.

Management/Treatment

Parenteral penicillin G is the only effective treatment for congenital syphilis. (6)(15) *T pallidum* has shown no resistance to penicillin, which has proved to be effective in maintaining the minimal concentration needed for treponemicidal levels over the treatment period. The frequency of penicillin dosing depends on age due to renal clearance because the serum half-life of penicillin G correlates inversely with age. (6)(16) Current treatment for infants older than 1 month is aqueous crystalline penicillin G 200,000 to 300,000 U/kg per day, intravenously administered as 50,000 U/kg every 4 to 6 hours for 10 days. (6)

Awareness of the Jarisch-Herxheimer reaction is important. Most commonly seen during treatment of primary and secondary seropositive syphilis, this reaction is due to a release of endotoxinlike antigens during bacterial lysis on starting penicillin. (3)(17) Symptoms include fever, hypotension, hyperventilation, headache, flushing, and vomiting. There is a reported increased risk with higher RPR titers (≥1:32). (18) Mild reactions are self-limiting and may resolve within the first 24 hours. Symptoms can usually be treated with only antipyretics or intravenous fluids if there is vital sign instability. If necessary, corticosteroids, vasopressors, or inotropic support may be used. This is not a contraindication to continuing treatment. (3)(18)

Table. Sensitivity and Specificity of Nontreponemal and Treponemal Testing in Primary Syphilis (13)(14)(19)

SYPHILIS TEST	SENSITIVITY, %	SPECIFICITY, %
Nontreponemal		
RPR	77–99	93–99
VDRL	74–87	96–99
Treponemal		
FTA-Abs	78.2–100	87–100
TP-PA	86.2–100	99.6–100
CIA	84.9–98.9	93.0–97.3
Treponema pallidum EIA	84.9–98.9	78.4–86.1

Note: The sensitivity and specificity vary based on time since infection. Abbreviations: CIA=chemiluminescence immunoassay, EIA=enzyme immunoassay, FTA-Abs=fluorescent treponemal antibody absorption, RPR=rapid plasma reagin, TP-PA=*Treponema pallidum* particle agglutination assay.

After initial treatment, patients with congenital syphilis should be followed every 2 to 3 months for repeated nontreponemal VDRL or RPR testing until it is nonreactive. The serologic response to treatment is often slower in infants diagnosed and treated beyond the neonatal period. However, should the patient continue to remain positive 12 months after treatment, repeated evaluation, including CSF examination, and repeated treatment with 10 days of parenteral penicillin G may be indicated. (6)

Lessons for the Clinician

- Syphilis can yield a negative test result if the mother is infected late in the pregnancy because treponemal assays take 3 to 4 weeks and nontreponemal assays take 4 to 6 weeks to detect antibodies.
- Consider syphilis for any rash involving the palms and soles with unknown etiology even if the history seems to be reassuring (eg, negative maternal prenatal syphilis testing).
- A Jarisch-Herxheimer reaction can occur during initiation of treatment with penicillin, usually resolves within the first 24 hours, and is not an indication for stopping treatment.
- After treatment for congenital syphilis, patients should be followed closely with repeated rapid plasma reagin titers every 2 to 3 months until their titer becomes nonreactive.

References for this article can be found at https://doi.org/10.1542/pir.2021-005372.

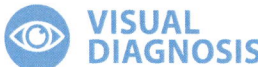

VISUAL DIAGNOSIS

Vulvar Ulcers in a Non–Sexually Active Adolescent

Alisa Corrado, MD,* Savannah Cheo, MD,* Rose Walczak, MD*

*Department of Pediatrics, Rush University Medical Center, Chicago, IL

PRESENTATION

A 16-year-old girl with no significant medical history presents with 5 days of vulvar pain and dysuria. She endorses a constant, sharp, burning labial pain. She has been febrile intermittently, with an initial maximum temperature of 103°F (39.4°C) 2 days earlier. She has been nauseous and experienced 1 episode of nonbloody, nonbilious emesis yesterday. Due to fear of urination, she has stopped eating and drinking the past 2 days. She has been using acetaminophen and ibuprofen every 6 to 8 hours for the past 5 days with no improvement in pain. She denies vaginal discharge, hematuria, urinary urgency or frequency, any sexual activity or trauma, new body products, or douching. She denies a history of arthralgias, rash, fatigue, hematochezia, visual changes, weight loss, recent upper respiratory tract infection symptoms, or recent vaccinations. Her menstrual periods come regularly every 28 days and last approximately 4 days. The first day of her last menstrual period was 2 days ago, and she is actively menstruating. She endorses a history of oral "cold sores" but denies previous genital lesions. Family history is negative, including no family history of autoimmune processes.

She has been seen by her primary care physician twice and in an emergency department once this week, diagnosed each time with a suspected urinary tract infection or yeast infection. Before admission, an initial complete blood cell count and complete metabolic panel in the emergency department were normal, and a urine pregnancy test was negative. A urinalysis in the emergency department was notable for amber color and a specific gravity of 1.028, protein level of 100 mg/dL, greater than 80 mg/dL ketones, positive nitrites, large blood, large leukocyte esterase, white blood cell count greater than 200 WBC/hpf, red blood cell count greater than 200 RBC/hpf, positive bilirubin, and moderate bacteria. However, urine culture data from these visits show no bacterial growth. She has now completed 2 days of cefalexin therapy, 2 days of metronidazole therapy, 1 day of nitrofurantoin therapy, and 1 dose of fluconazole. She was also prescribed trimethoprim/sulfamethoxazole but has not taken it yet. None of these antimicrobial agents, or phenazopyridine, have relieved the pain.

Vital signs on presentation are notable for tachycardia to the low 100s beats/min. She is otherwise afebrile, normotensive, and has a normal respiratory rate and oxygen saturation on room air. She has dry mucous membranes, but no oral lesions are noted. Genital examination is pertinent for bilateral, shallow, tender vaginal ulcerations along the labia minora and vaginal introitus, as well as edema of the labia majora (Fig 1). There is no visible discharge or bleeding or any perianal lesions. A pelvic examination is deferred due to patient discomfort. Examination is not notable for inguinal lymphadenopathy.

AUTHOR DISCLOSURE: Drs Corrado, Cheo, and Walczak have disclosed no financial relationships relevant to this article. This commentary does not contain a discussion of an unapproved/investigative use of a commercial product/device.

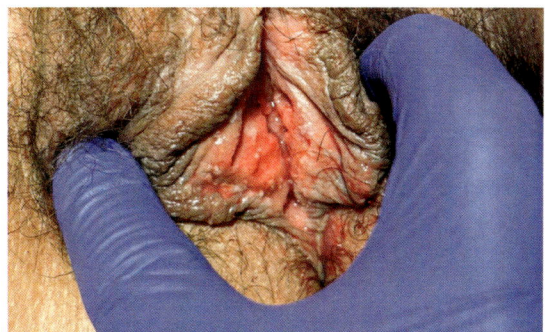

Figure 1. Vulvar ulcerations on arrival.

Due to the need for intravenous pain control and Foley catheter placement for urination (Fig 2), the patient is admitted to the hospital. Gynecology and rheumatology are consulted on arrival at the general pediatrics floor, recommending a full laboratory evaluation for sexually transmitted infections. Testing for chlamydia, gonorrhea, trichomonas, human immunodeficiency virus, syphilis, bacterial vaginosis, and yeast are unrevealing. Polymerase chain reaction (PCR) testing for herpes simplex virus (HSV) types 1 and 2 was negative. There is low concern for a systemic autoimmune process, such as Bechet disease or systemic lupus erythematosus, given the lack of other features on history/clinical examination, including pathergy, oral ulcers, eye or brain involvement, joint involvement, lack of recurrent symptoms, and lack of typical ethnicity. Similar, "knife-life" ulcerations can be seen with cutaneous Crohn disease. However, inflammatory bowel disease is deemed less likely given her lack of gastrointestinal symptoms.

Dermatology is also consulted, recommending antibody titers for Epstein-Barr virus (EBV), cytomegalovirus, and

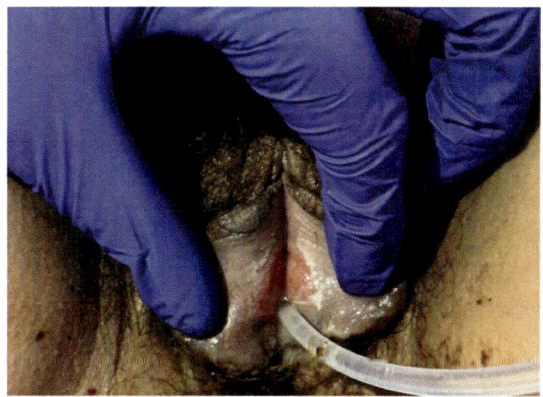

Figure 2. Vulvar ulcerations on hospital day 2, with Foley placement.

mycoplasma. This infectious evaluation is significant for EBV IgG elevation to 3.2 Ab index, and an EBV nuclear capsid antibody elevation to 63.3 U/mL (positive result >21 U/mL). The patient's history and examination findings confirm the diagnosis.

DIAGNOSIS

The patient was diagnosed as having Lipschutz ulcers, also known as non–sexually acquired genital ulceration.

DISCUSSION

Genital ulcers, although less common in pediatrics than in the adult population, have an annual global incidence estimated near 20 million cases. When considering the etiology of genital ulcers, one may first investigate infectious, which are more common, followed by noninfectious causes. (1) The most common infectious causes (in order of frequency) are genital HSV-1/2, syphilis, chancroid (although rates have vastly declined in the United States in the past decade), lymphogranuloma venereum, granuloma inguinale (donovanosis), fungal infection such as candida, or a secondary bacterial infection of preexisting trauma. The most common noninfectious causes include Behcet syndrome, fixed drug eruptions, psoriasis, sexual trauma, and Wegener granulomatosis. (1) Less common causes of noninfectious genital ulcers to consider also include inflammatory bowel disease and other autoimmune processes, such as systemic lupus erythematosus.

Lipschutz ulcers, although often described as an immunologic response to infection or inflammation, are a noninfectious etiology of genital ulcers most commonly found in non–sexually active women younger than 20 years. (2) The exact prevalence is unknown. Symptoms typically begin with prodromal flulike symptoms, followed by the appearance of 1 to 3 large (>10 mm), well-demarcated, painful vulvar ulcerations in a "mirrorlike" distribution. (2)(3) They are often accompanied by labial edema. (4) Dysuria to the point of requiring catheterization is relatively common, affecting nearly 10% of documented Lipschutz cases. (2) Inguinal lymphadenopathy, although not observed in this patient, can also accompany ulcerations in close to 10% of cases. (2)

The most commonly associated infections include (in order of frequency) EBV, mycoplasma, cytomegalovirus, and influenza. (2) Recently, cases of vulvar aphthous ulcers after COVID-19 infection and vaccination have also been reported. (5) This rare diagnosis is one of exclusion, namely, of the aforementioned infectious and rheumatologic causes of similar presentations. Evaluation should entail skin swabs for PCR testing and culture. PCR remains the most sensitive and specific testing modality for HSV-1/2. Biopsy tends to be traumatic, and findings are nonspecific. (4)

Lipschutz ulcers tend to resolve without recurrence or scarring within 3 weeks, with approximately 10% of cases lasting longer than 1 month. (2) Treatment typically includes reassurance, local hygiene and removal of irritating factors (such as tight clothing or scented soaps or panty liners), wound care, and pain control. (2)(4) Topical corticosteroids are useful for pain control and facilitating healing. A recent systematic review of Lipschutz ulcers did not support the use of systemic corticosteroids in treatment because disease duration was shorter in patients who did not receive systemic corticosteroids. However, this review did not account for clinical severity of disease. (2) Although topical lidocaine 5% ointment was not used in this case, it remains a safe and viable option for local pain control in vulvar ulcerations.

PATIENT COURSE

This patient had a severe course that required a several-day admission for pain control, requiring intravenous morphine. Per dermatology recommendations, she was started on systemic prednisone 0.5 mg/kg once daily and 2.5% topical hydrocortisone ointment twice daily. She required intravenous fluid resuscitation and Foley placement to maintain normal urination while the systemic corticosteroids facilitated healing. She was discharged on hospital day 4 with resolution of her pain using naproxen, prednisone, and topical hydrocortisone. Her lesions were nearly completely resolved by her 1-week follow-up appointment with the pediatrician and have not since recurred.

Summary

- Lipschutz ulcers should be considered when young, non–sexually active females present with painful vaginal ulcerations. They may be associated with labial edema, dysuria, and inguinal lymphadenopathy.

- Lipschutz ulcers are a diagnosis of exclusion and should be considered after more common causes of vaginal ulceration (both infectious and noninfectious) have been ruled out.

- The treatment of Lipschutz ulcers is mainly supportive care and pain control. Topical corticosteroids (and even systemic corticosteroids) may be beneficial in healing; however, further randomized controlled trials are warranted to investigate efficacy.

- Nearly all Lipschutz ulcers resolve within 4 weeks of onset without recurrence or long-term sequelae.

References for this article can be found at
https://doi.org/10.1542/pir.2022-005917.

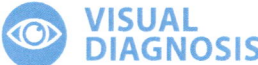

Healthy Infant with Numerous Yellow Papules

Malina Yamashita Peterson, MD,* Alexis J. Lukach, MD,† Sarah Asch, MD‡

*Gundersen Lutheran Medical Center, La Crosse, WI
†Yardley Dermatology Associates, Yardley, PA
‡Hometown Pediatric Dermatology PLLC, North Oaks, MN

PRESENTATION

An 8-month-old healthy boy presents to the dermatology clinic with a 3-month history of increasingly numerous skin papules. On review of systems, the patient has a history of a single episode of atraumatic brief swelling of the hand that self-resolved. There is no history of fever, weight change, or relatives or close contacts with similar papules. Physical examination reveals a well-appearing interactive male infant. Full-body skin examination shows approximately 100 smooth, firm, 1- to 15-mm yellow-pink papules and nodules that are scattered on the head and concentrated on the trunk, genitals, and buttocks (Fig 1). When the lesions are stroked, they do not urticate (Darier sign). A few of the larger lesions are umbilicated. He does not have hepatosplenomegaly. The dermatologist performs a punch biopsy. Given the extent of cutaneous findings, additional evaluation is performed. Results of ophthalmologic examination, abdominal ultrasonography, complete blood cell counts, and liver function tests are within normal limits. However, his skeletal survey reveals multiple lytic and sclerotic lesions (Fig 2), and the patient is referred to pediatric hematology/oncology. There is no functional compromise or sign of other internal organ involvement. Results of the punch biopsy confirm the diagnosis.

DIAGNOSIS

The differential diagnosis for numerous pink-yellow papules in a well-appearing infant includes Langerhans cell histiocytosis (LCH), Spitz nevi, and molluscum contagiosum. LCH is typically more scaly with smaller papules and surrounding dermatitis and is more similar in appearance to seborrheic dermatitis. (1) Spitz nevi are less likely as these benign pediatric neoplasms are usually solitary and rarely eruptive-disseminated. (2) Although molluscum contagiosum is a common disease, it is less common in a young infant. (3) Molluscum contagiosum lesions also tend to surface and resolve, and a few lesions are typically umbilicated. (3) In addition, severe molluscum contagiosum in an infant raises concern for immune deficiency; however, the patient has no previous infections and is growing well. (3)

A punch biopsy reveals a brisk dermal proliferation of CD68-positive, S100-negative foamy histiocytes with interspersed Touton giant cells (Fig 3). He is diagnosed as having systemic juvenile xanthogranuloma (JXG).

AUTHOR DISCLOSURE: Ms Peterson and Drs Lukach and Asch have disclosed no financial relationships relevant to this article. This commentary does not contain a discussion of an unapproved/investigative use of a commercial product/device.

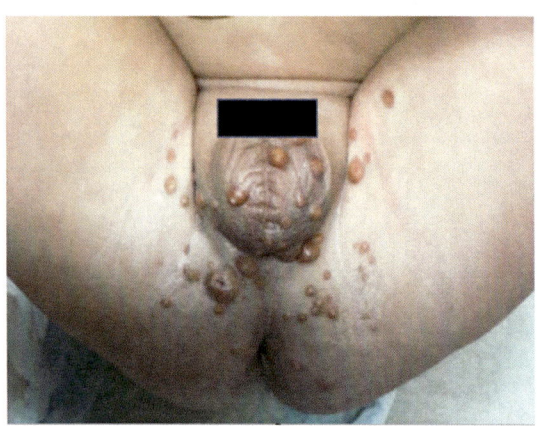

Figure 1. Numerous shiny, firm, 1- to 15-mm, pink-yellow papules and nodules in the groin, with a few larger lesions showing umbilication. Similar lesions are concentrated on the trunk and scattered on the head and neck.

DISCUSSION

JXG is the most common type of non-LCH and is classically characterized by 0.5- to 2.0-cm firm, round, tan-yellow papules or nodules. These asymptomatic lesions present early in life and typically regress within 3 to

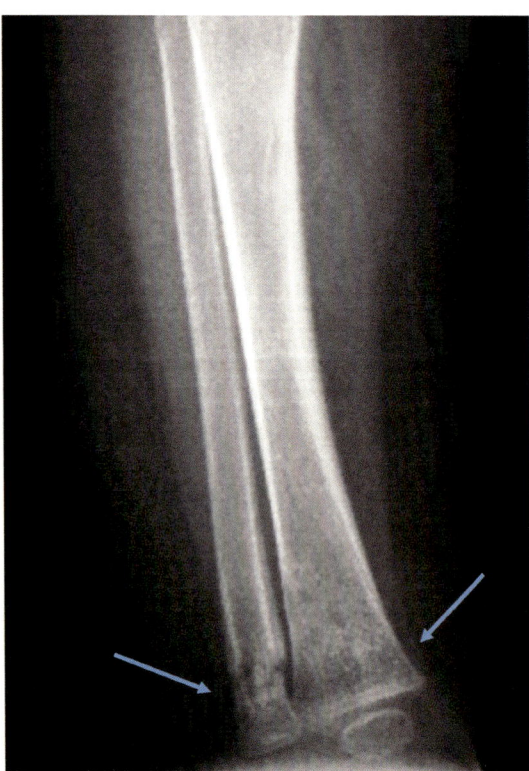

Figure 2. Lytic lesions and periosteal bony reaction, evidenced by patchy areas of lucency (arrows), of the distal metadiaphysis of the right fibula and tibia.

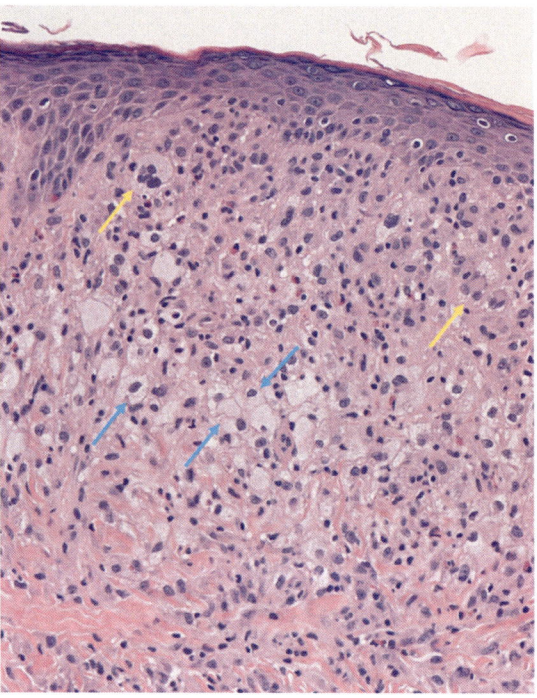

Figure 3. Lymphohistiocytic dermal infiltrate of foamy histiocytes, as well as scattered multinucleated and Touton giant cells (H&E, ×20). Histiocytes can typically be recognized by their relatively large size, eccentric nuclei, and foamy cytoplasm (blue arrows). Multinucleated giant cells are visualized exactly as their name suggests, and Touton giant cells are a subtype where the nuclei form a ring on the periphery of the cell (yellow arrows).

6 years. (4) In retrospective analysis of reported cases, 34.5% of cases are congenital, (5) and up to 79% of cases are diagnosed within the first year after birth. (4)(6) Presentation beyond early childhood is less common, with 2.9% of reported cases diagnosed between 16 and 20 years old. (6)

JXG can present with single or multiple lesions. Studies show that more than 80% of patients with JXG present with a solitary lesion. (5)(6) Most patients with multiple JXG present with 10 lesions or less. (4) Similar to isolated JXG, multiple JXG most commonly involves the head and neck, trunk, extremities, and gluteal region, but it can present as scattered, linear, lichenoid, agminated or segmental, and micronodular and macronodular. (4) Given that systemic involvement is more common with multiple JXGs, and the differential diagnosis includes LCH, agminated Spitz nevus, molluscum, or infections; biopsy confirms the diagnosis and the need for systemic evaluation.

Systemic JXG is defined by the presence of a JXG at an extracutaneous site. Systemic disease is rare with a single cutaneous lesion, occurring in only approximately 7% of cases; in contrast, 38.2% of patients with multiple skin lesions have involvement of 1 extracutaneous site and 19.3% have involvement of more than 1 extracutaneous site. (4) In patients with systemic JXG, the eye is the most commonly affected internal organ, followed by the liver and spleen, lung, kidney, central nervous system, and bone. (4)

Systemic JXG may result in complications. In retrospective reviews of reported cases, 4% to 5% of reported cases are systemic JXG. (5)(6) Serious complications from systemic JXG are uncommon and typically result from mass effect or invasion. Ocular JXG can cause secondary glaucoma or vision loss. (7) Liver JXG can lead to liver failure, coagulopathy, and electrolyte changes. (4)

JXG is often a clinical diagnosis. Dermatology referral can be useful for complete skin examination, biopsy, and coordinating referral for extracutaneous screening and management. Although the diagnosis is often clinical, pathology reveals a dense dermal histiocytic infiltrate with Touton giant cells, with immunohistochemical analysis positive for CD68 and negative for CD100 and CD1a. (8)

Physicians may consider screening for extracutaneous JXG. The screening for extracutaneous JXG should be tailored based on age, number of lesions, and symptoms and may include computed tomography and magnetic resonance imaging, complete blood cell count, comprehensive metabolic panel, and coagulation profile. A lipid profile is not indicated because JXG is a normolipemic process. (9) More comprehensive screening is recommended for patients younger than 3 years with more than 10 cutaneous lesions, and this screening should include abdominal ultrasonography and ophthalmologic examination. (4)(10) If systemic involvement is detected, patients should be referred to appropriate services, which most commonly include pediatric ophthalmology for eye involvement and pediatric hematology/oncology for bone or other organ involvement. (4)(10)

Treatment of systemic JXG may be needed only for symptomatic cases. Treatment of systemic JXG is only necessary when lesions compromise bodily functions or development because most lesions will spontaneously involute over time. (11) When required, treatment is case-dependent, using surgery for localized disease or systemic chemotherapy for severe generalized presentations. (9)(12)

The association of multiple cutaneous JXG with juvenile myelomonocytic leukemia and neurofibromatosis type 1 remains unclear. (4)(13) Current data do not support repeated laboratory testing to evaluate for juvenile myelomonocytic leukemia in the absence of fevers, unusual bruising, or hepatosplenomegaly. (4) However, a complete history and thorough review of systems should be obtained regularly.

PATIENT COURSE

This patient has extensive cutaneous JXG, prompting systemic evaluation. Systemic involvement consisting of isolated bone lesions is rare, occurring in less than 8% of cases. (4) At the time of diagnosis, several of the skeletal lesions demonstrate sclerosis, suggesting early stages of resolution. Given the already self-resolving course, our patient does not require systemic treatment. At his follow-up appointment, the patient continues to be in good health. He is toddler-age, and his skin lesions are either completely resolved or flattening. Follow-up radiography shows continued resolution of bony lesions. The patient continues to follow up with dermatology and pediatric hematology/oncology yearly until resolution.

Summary

- Juvenile xanthogranuloma (JXG) presents as 0.5- to 2.0-cm firm, round, tan-yellow papules or nodules that present in the first year after birth and typically regress within 3 to 6 years.

- Systemic involvement of JXG rarely occurs with single lesions. Clinical diagnosis is typical for single lesions; for multiple lesions there is a differential diagnosis that includes Langerhans cell histiocytosis, agminated Spitz nevus, molluscum, or infections, and it should be further evaluated.

- Comprehensive screening for extracutaneous JXG is recommended for patients younger than 3 years with more than 10 cutaneous lesions, and this screening should include abdominal ultrasonography and ophthalmologic examination. (1)

- Screening for ocular involvement should be performed for those younger than 2 years with multiple cutaneous lesions and for any number with ocular concerns. Patients presenting with ocular JXG should be screened for cutaneous JXG.

- Treatment of systemic JXG is necessary only when lesions compromise bodily functions or development.

References for this article can be found at
https://doi.org/10.1542/pir.2022-005601.

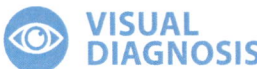

VISUAL DIAGNOSIS

Coral Fluorescing Axillary Plaques Refractory to Topical Antifungal and Antibacterial Treatments

Brendan P. Stewart, MD,* Kayla Gonzalez, MD,† Caleb Wasser, DO, FAAP‡

*UConn General Surgery Residency, University of Connecticut School of Medicine, Farmington, CT
†University of Connecticut Pediatrics Residency Program, Farmington, CT
‡Connecticut Children's Medical Center, Hartford, CT

PRESENTATION

An 8-year-old boy with a medical history significant for obesity (BMI, 34.75) and anxiety presents to the clinic with a bilateral axillary rash. The rash began under the right arm 2 months before presentation, and he simultaneously developed a similar, but less expansive, lesion in the left axilla. The rash is a 2- to 3-in (5.1- to 7.6-cm) circular plaque with beefy red coloration and raised macerated edges; the right axilla is worse than the left axilla. The patient is prescribed clotrimazole topical 1% cream for a presumed fungal infection to be applied twice a day and is advised to follow up in 1 month.

At the follow-up visit 1 month later, the patient is still experiencing the bilateral rash, which is now associated with pruritus. At this visit, the rash still appears as a beefy red color with overlying thick hyperkeratotic scaling and macerated edges. During this visit, the rash is examined under a Wood's lamp, which displays coral fluorescence (Fig 1). An aerobic skin culture is also performed at this visit. The patient is prescribed topical clindamycin for a presumed bacterial infection or erythrasma, and follow-up is scheduled in the clinic in 2 weeks.

Two weeks later the patient presents with continued rash that is still itchy. The aerobic skin culture, collected at the previous visit, grew heavy growth of methicillin-sensitive *Staphylococcus aureus*. The patient reports using no new lotions or creams and that the rash is slightly improving. On examination the patient still has the bilateral erythematous rash appearing as circular plaques with hyperkeratotic scales on the outer edges, which remains fluorescent under the Wood's lamp. The patient is prescribed an additional week of topical clindamycin gel and is instructed to return in 1 week.

One week later, he presents with a worsening rash. The right axilla now has surrounding erythematous macular skin irritation, and the initial plaque is still beefy red with hyperkeratotic scaling and macerated edges that fluoresces under a Wood's lamp (Fig 2). Because the topical antibiotic ointment was ineffective, the patient is treated with oral erythromycin and referred to a dermatologist. Two weeks later, the patient presents to dermatology with the initial plaques surrounded by expanding erythematous urticarial papules associated with pruritus. The patient undergoes two 4-mm skin punch biopsies at sites 1 and 2 in the left axilla (Fig 3). Site 1 histopathology shows orthohyperkeratosis, parakeratosis, neutrophils, and serum in the stratum corneum; neutrophils in the upper epidermis; hypogranulosis; pseudocarcinomatous epidermal hyperplasia; thinning of suprapapillary plates; dilated and tortuous vessels in the papillary epidermis; and superficial, perivascular, and interstitial infiltrate of

AUTHOR DISCLOSUURE: Drs Stewart, Gonzalez, and Wasser have disclosed no financial relationships relevant to this article. This commentary does not contain a discussion of an unapproved/investigative use of a commercial product/device.

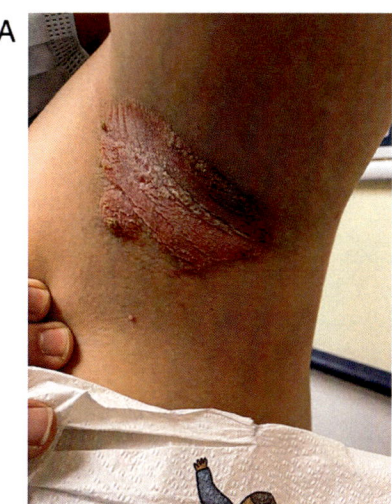 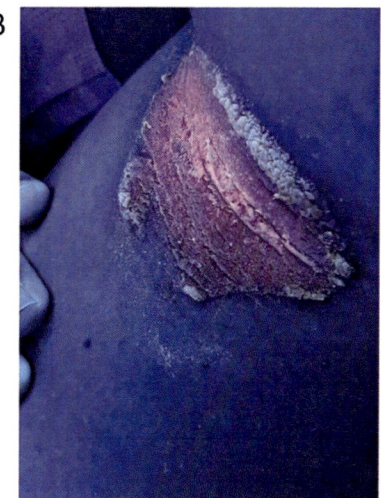

Figure 1. The patient's left axilla before treatment with topical clindamycin seen under normal light (A) and Wood's lamp (B).

lymphocytes, histiocytes, and neutrophils. Immunostaining for human papillomavirus types 6, 11, 16, 18, 31, 33, 42, 51, 52, 56, and 58 is negative. Periodic acid–Schiff stain for fungal elements and Gram-stain for bacteria are negative. Site 2 histopathology showed parakeratosis, epidermal acanthosis, and subcorneal collections of neutrophils with a superficial and mid-dermal infiltrate of lymphocytes, histiocytes, and neutrophils. Gram-stain and periodic acid–Schiff stain were also negative at site 2. Histopathology confirms the diagnosis.

DIAGNOSIS

Based on review of the histopathologic findings from the skin punch biopsies and clinical assessment, a final diagnosis of inverse psoriasis is made.

DISCUSSION

On initial presentation, common diagnoses to be considered for plaques of this nature include fungal intertrigo, bacterial (erythrasma), psoriasis, eczema, and granular parakeratosis. Fungal etiologies were less likely after there was no improvement with clotrimazole treatment. Our suspicion for dermatitis was low given no history, lack of lichenified lesions with excoriations, and the overall size and thickness of the plaques on presentation. (1) Granular parakeratosis was also considered; however, the patient had no recent changes in deodorants, lotions, soaps, or other possible irritants, which made us less likely to consider this reaction as an etiology of the patient's presenting symptoms. (2) Our leading diagnoses were erythrasma

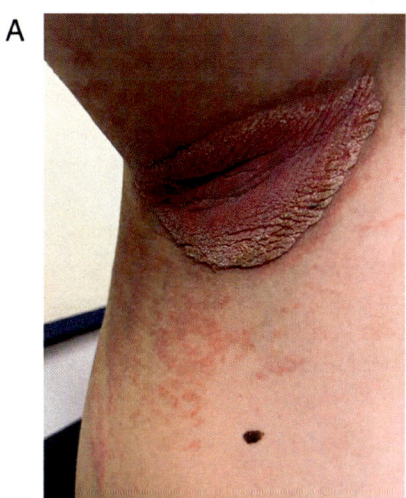 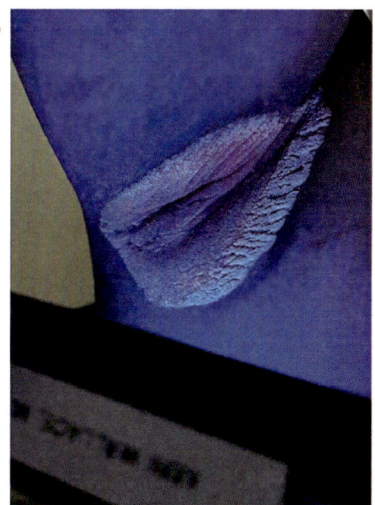

Figure 2. The patient's right axilla after treatment with topical clindamycin. A. Beefy-red, macerated, hyperkeratotic scaling seen under normal light. B. Coral-red fluorescence visualized under Wood's lamp.

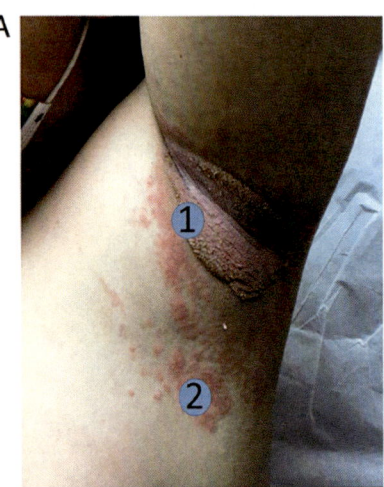
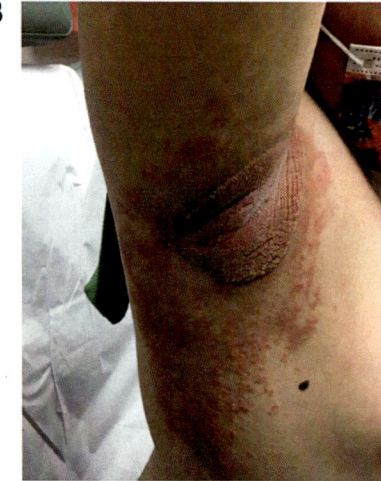

Figure 3. The patient's left and right axillae after treatment with oral erythromycin and topical clindamycin. A. The patient's left axilla with circles marked 1 and 2 indicating the 2 locations of skin biopsies. B. The patient's right axilla.

and psoriasis. However, after both topical and oral antibiotics were ineffective, we considered erythrasma less likely despite our Wood's lamp findings. In addition, our patient did not display signs of systemic psoriasis and inflammation, such as nail pitting, inflammatory bowel disease, diabetes, or arthritic pains, which would have helped cement a diagnosis of psoriasis. (3) This leaves the most likely diagnosis as an abnormal presentation of psoriasis.

Psoriasis and erythrasma are commonly included together in the differential diagnosis of plaquelike lesions similar to our patient. (4) Psoriasis is an inflammatory skin disease found in approximately 1% of children, with the most typical onset being around 7 to 10 years of age. (5) In the pediatric population, psoriasis is most commonly found on the scalp, face, trunk, and extremities. (5) Compared with the adult population, plaque psoriasis in pediatrics is usually less scaly and not as thick. (5) Inverse psoriasis, as present in our patient, is a subclass of psoriasis commonly located around skin folds. (6) Numerous risk factors have been proposed for developing psoriasis, including stress and skin trauma. (5) Obesity has also been the focus of recent research as a comorbidity of psoriasis, with obesity being associated with more severe psoriasis. (5) Various medications have also been linked to causing a psoriasiform drug reaction, including β-blockers, lithium, and antimalarial medications. In addition, note that a diagnosis of psoriasis is more commonly made in patients with lighter skin types compared with patients with darker skin types. (7)

Erythrasma is a skin condition most commonly caused by *Corynebacterium minutissimum*. (8) More commonly seen in adult populations, erythrasma is rare in the pediatric population. (9) Erythrasma is frequently located in the axillary

or inguinal regions, and there is increased risk for individuals who are obese or diabetic. (8–11) Additional risk factors predisposing patients to erythrasma infections include male sex, hot/humid climates, and living in populated areas such as college dormitories. (8) Our patient presented with an obese body habitus and a BMI of 34.75, putting him at risk for both psoriasis and erythrasma. He presented in December through March in the Northeast, ruling out climate as a contributing factor. In addition, he lived at home with his parents and sibling with no pets. There was no report of new medications or trauma to the bilateral axilla.

Despite resembling fungal infections such as candidiasis or dermatophyte infection, dermatitis, or inflammatory reactions such as psoriasis, a diagnosis of erythrasma and psoriasis can made via examination with a Wood's lamp. Erythrasma will exhibit characteristic coral-red fluorescence under the blue light due to production of porphyrins by *C minutissimum*. (8, 11, 12) Although it has also been historically reported that psoriasis will display a similar red fluorescent color under Wood's lamp, in more recent studies, patients with inverse psoriasis with fluorescence under Wood's lamp has been attributed to erythrasma. (13, 14) However, note that psoriasis can present differently depending on the patient's skin color. In patients with lighter skin types, psoriasis will present with more pink/red hues, whereas patients with darker skin types present with lesions of more violaceous pigmentation. (7)

As evident in Figs 1 and 2, our patient's lesions displayed coral-red fluorescence under the Wood's lamp in both axillae. A definitive diagnosis of erythrasma can be determined with a skin biopsy or culture, which will show Gram-positive coccobacilli in the stratum corneum, the most superficial dermal layer. (9, 11, 15) Skin cultures should be performed if the Wood's lamp evaluation is inconclusive and the clinician still suspects a bacterial infection. (16) On the other hand, if a clinician is suspecting psoriasis, diagnosis is most often made from clinical scoring systems; skin biopsy is rarely required. (17) However, biopsy is definitive, and histopathology will display hyperkeratosis, parakeratosis, elongated epidermal ridges, dilated blood vessels in the dermis, and inflammatory infiltrates in the dermis and epidermis. (17) Skin biopsies are typically indicated when there is suspicion for a serious condition, when diagnosis cannot be made in a less-invasive manner, when treatment will be guided based on histopathologic findings, or when a patient fails to respond to initial therapies. (18) With our patient, the decision was made to also test the biopsy samples for human papillomavirus immunostaining given the hyperkeratotic nature of the lesion on biopsy. (19)

Erythrasma can be treated with topical or oral antibiotics, with macrolides serving as the treatment of choice. (11) Clarithromycin and erythromycin, both macrolides, and clindamycin, a lincosamide, have all been used as treatments. (11, 15, 16, 20) These are bacteriostatic antibiotics that inhibit the 50s subunit of bacterial ribosomes, preventing protein translation and synthesis. (21) Topical macrolides are commonly preferred to prevent adverse effects, including gastrointestinal complaints such as nausea, vomiting, and diarrhea; cardiac effects such as prolonged QT interval; and cutaneous reactions such as Stevens-Johnson syndrome or toxic epidermal necrolysis. (21, 22) Most recently, fusidic acid and mupirocin have been used with success in treating erythrasma. Mupirocin inhibits protein synthesis by binding to isoleucyl-tRNA synthesis and inhibiting protein synthesis, and fusidic acid binds elongation factor G and inhibits protein synthesis. (8, 11, 12, 23, 24) Treatment of erythrasma has proved to be difficult, with infection commonly recurring after a full course of antibiotics. (8, 11)

Our patient had failed initial therapy with topical clindamycin and oral erythromycin, and we ultimately decided to refer him for a biopsy. The biopsy of the main plaques was negative for stains of any bacteria or fungal component and more closely resembled the histologic description of psoriasis. No culture was sent of the samples; however, given that the patient was treated with both topical and oral antibiotics, it is possible that there were no viable bacteria on the lesions at the time of biopsy. The initial skin swab for our patient did not show results consistent with *C minutissimum* on Gram-stain but did show heavy growth of methicillin-sensitive *S aureus*, which has been shown to be associated with psoriasis. (25)

Psoriasis, as well as inverse psoriasis, in both the adult and pediatric populations is initially treated with topical therapies,

including topical glucocorticoids. (5, 17) Topical corticosteroids are not without harm, and common adverse effects that must be considered include skin atrophy, acne, skin infections, and changes in pigmentation. (5, 17, 26) In addition, UV light has additionally been proved as a treatment for psoriasis; however, safety in pediatric patient populations is still lacking. (27, 28) Absolute contraindications to UV therapy include systemic lupus erythematosus, basal cell nevus syndrome, and xeroderma pigmentosum, and relative contraindications include history of skin cancers, photosensitivity disorders, and use for psoriasis in the genital areas. (28–30)

Last, note that histopathology showed secondary subcorneal pustular dermatitis as satellite lesions surrounding the hyperkeratotic plaques in our patient at biopsy site 2. Given that these lesions appeared after treatment with oral erythromycin, a possible cause is a drug reaction that has been reported after the use of topical clindamycin and oral erythromycin. (22, 31, 32) However, it is also possible that the satellite lesions were from progression of the psoriasis. For the previously stated reasons, we believe that the patient was experiencing inverse psoriasis complicated with probable erythrasma, which resolved with topical treatments.

PATIENT COURSE

The patient reported that the rash fully resolved bilaterally on administration of triamcinolone 0.1%. Because our patient did not display signs of systemic inflammation, topical treatments were solely used as opposed to systemic therapies. On cessation of topical treatment, the rash began to recur in both axillae. Due to recurrence, the patient was prescribed triamcinolone 0.1% to use for 2 weeks for eruptions as needed with maintenance treatment of tacrolimus 0.03% topical cream to use twice daily.

Summary

- This case highlights the role of skin biopsies to differentiate between inflammatory and microbial causes of plaques that may appear similar even under UV Wood's lamp examination.

- Especially with pediatric rashes, it is important to consider both the presenting symptoms and the patient's risk factors and comorbid conditions to help elucidate the underlying cause.

- If a patient does not respond to medications to treat the initial diagnosis, a broader differential diagnosis should be considered.

References for this article can be found at
https://doi.org/10.1542/pir.2022-005770.

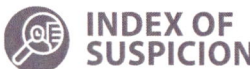

INDEX OF SUSPICION

Sun-Induced Rash in a 6-year-old Girl

David A. Shafique, MD,* Aeja N. Weiss, MD,† Shannan E. McCann, MD†

*United States Air Force, Shaw AFB, SC
†United States Air Force, Lackland AFB, TX

PRESENTATION

A healthy 6-year-old girl, Fitzpatrick skin type V (see Table 1 for classification [1]), with a history of atopic dermatitis and seasonal allergies presents with 3 years of a transient, recurrent, summertime rash on her face and neck. The rash is not painful, itchy, or associated with other systemic symptoms. It typically occurs 24 to 48 hours after her first visit to the pool each summer independent of swimming or sunscreen use. She tried treatment with emollients and hydrocortisone 1% cream without improvement. The rash lasts several weeks before resolving spontaneously without scarring or pigment changes.

The patient's medications include cetirizine, a multivitamin, and probiotic gummies. She has no known medication allergies or previous exposure to new soaps, detergents, fragrances, skin care products, or other potential triggers. Her family history is normal, with no history of autoimmune conditions or connective tissue disorders. No family members, friends, or other close contacts have similar symptoms.

The patient is well-appearing, and her vital signs, growth, and development are within normal limits. Examination demonstrates numerous 1- to 2-mm monomorphic, asymptomatic, skin-colored papules predominantly photodistributed on her central face, posterior neck, upper back, upper chest, and proximal upper extremities (Fig 1). A striking absence of lesions in the distribution of a bathing suit is noted. The hands, feet, nails, and mucosa are spared. Pinhead-sized, skin-colored papules arranged in 2 straight lines along the patient's right lateral elbow are identified (Fig 2).

DISCUSSION

Differential Diagnosis

Given the patient's overall good health, the strong association of her rash with sun exposure, and the clear photodistribution of lesions, common photodermatoses were considered in the differential diagnosis (Table 2). (2) This is not a comprehensive list of photosensitivity disorders, as more rare photodermatoses secondary to systemic disease, vitamin deficiency, and disorders of DNA repair are not included. In addition, nonphotosensitive conditions presenting with widespread papules such as miliaria, keratosis pilaris, molluscum contagiosum, and papular eczema were considered but are not discussed.

Polymorphous light eruption (PMLE) is a response to UV radiation (UVR) resulting in papules, vesicles, plaques, or eczematous eruptions within hours to days after exposure to sunlight. (2) In children, PMLE frequently begins on the face with an acute erythematous and eczematous dermatitis with small papules

AUTHOR DISCLOSURE: Drs Shafique, Weiss, and McCann have disclosed no financial relationships relevant to this article. This commentary does not contain a discussion of an unapproved/investigative use of a commercial product/device.

Disclaimer: The views expressed are those of the authors and do not reflect the official views or policies of the Department of Defense or its components.

Table 1. Fitzpatrick Skin Phototypes (1)

FITZPATRICK SKIN TYPE	PHENOTYPE	SKIN REACTION
I	White skin	Always burns, never tans
II	Fair skin	Usually burns, tans less than average
III	Darker white skin	Sometimes burns (mild), average tanning
IV	Light brown skin	Burns minimally, tans more than average
V	Brown skin	Rarely burns, tans deeply
VI	Dark brown or black skin	Never burns, tans deeply

in late spring and early summer. (2) Skin findings are typically pruritic and resolve without scarring within several days to weeks. PMLE can be associated with nonspecific systemic symptoms, such as malaise, chills, headache, and nausea.

Patients with systemic lupus erythematosus may develop a PMLE-like reaction. (3) These lesions appear and resolve more quickly than in PMLE, occurring immediately after sun exposure and often resolving within 1 day. (3) Up to 70% of patients with cutaneous lupus erythematosus (CLE) demonstrate photosensitivity. (3) The classic rash of acute CLE is malar erythema that spares the nasolabial folds, although a generalized morbilliform eruption may be observed. (4) Nearly 100% of patients with acute CLE will develop systemic lupus erythematosus. (4)

Juvenile spring eruption is considered a subtype of PMLE. (5) It presents in childhood or adolescence as erythematous, scaly papules or bullae on the helices of the ears but can involve the face, trunk, and dorsal hands. Males are affected more frequently than females, and lesions resolve within several weeks without recurrence until the following year. (5)

Actinic prurigo presents with intensely pruritic lesions of the face and arms (sometimes extending onto sun-protected skin) that last into the winter. (6) It most commonly affects Native Americans, especially those of Mestizo descent. (7) Pruritic papules, nodules, and plaques with excoriations and crusting often become lichenified and heal with scarring. (2)(6) A distinguishing feature seen in 33% to 85% of patients is actinic cheilitis, which presents with itch, pain, and tingling of the vermillion lip. (8)(9) Conjunctival involvement is found in up to 45% of patients. (6)(10)

Solar urticaria causes an itchy, burning sensation that develops into erythematous wheals within minutes of exposure to UVR or visible light. (2) Lesions resolve within hours as opposed to days with PMLE. These patients can have associated light-headedness, nausea, bronchospasm, malaise, and syncope.

Hydroa vacciniforme appears within hours of sun exposure as burning or pruritic erythematous macules that progress to

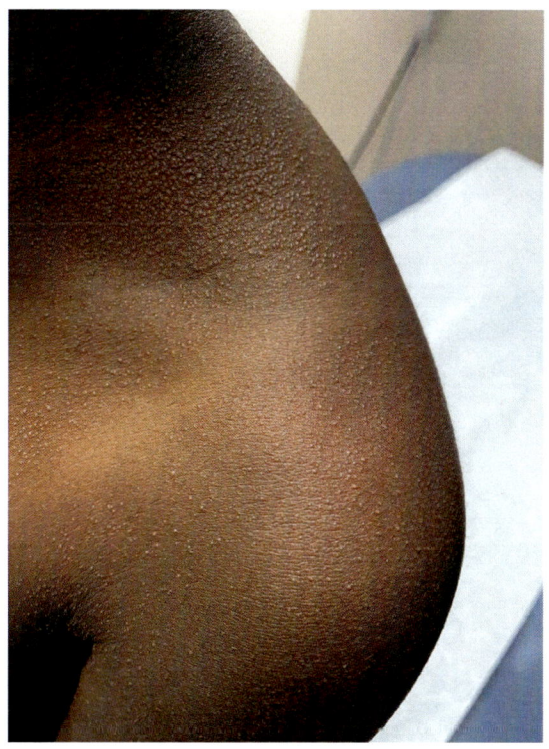

Figure 1. Diffuse, monomorphic, skin-colored papules of the left shoulder and left lateral neck with sparing of the skin covered by a bathing suit strap.

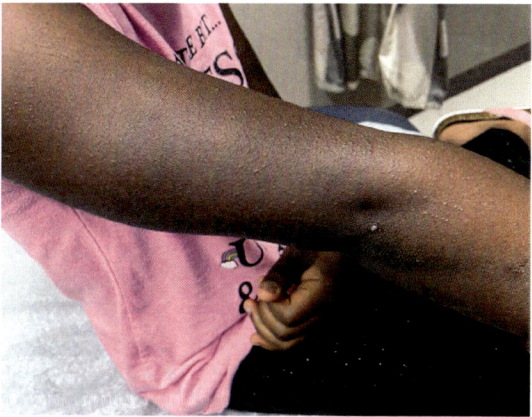

Figure 2. Two linear lesions superficial to the right lateral epicondyle secondary to the trauma from scratching (Koebner phenomenon).

Table 2. Differential Diagnosis for Common Photodermatoses (2)

- Polymorphous light eruption
- Actinic prurigo
- Juvenile spring eruption
- Solar urticaria
- Hydroa vacciniforme
- Phytophotodermatitis
- Phototoxicity
- Photoallergy
- Porphyrias (erythropoietic protoporphyria, porphyria cutanea tarda, congenital erythropoietic porphyria, hepatoerythropoietic porphyria, variegate porphyria, and hereditary coproporphyria)
- Systemic lupus erythematosus

tender papules, vesicles, and crusts that heal with depressed scars. (2) Preceding infection with Epstein-Barr virus infection has been associated with hydroa vacciniforme, and elevated levels of Epstein-Barr virus DNA have been detected in patients with active skin lesions. (11)

Phototoxicity results from direct injury to cells after UVR exposure when photoreactive chemicals are transformed into cytotoxic products. (12) The damage to skin cells usually occurs within hours after exposure to an offending agent and presents like an exaggerated sunburn with burning erythema and edema. When severe, vesicles and bullae can develop. (2) Table 3 contains common culprits. (12)(13) Phytophotodermatitis is a type of phototoxicity that results after skin comes into contact with plant-derived, light-sensitizing compounds (furocoumarins). Areas of skin that contact both furocoumarins and UVR develop erythema, edema, or vesicles. (14) Phytophotodermatitis heals with hyperpigmentation, which fades over weeks to months.

Photoallergy is a delayed-type hypersensitivity reaction to an allergen that changes antigenicity after exposure to UVR. Previous sensitization to the photoallergen (or one that cross-reacts with it) is required, and skin changes appear after 24 to 48 hours. Pruritic, eczematous eruptions occur in regions of sun-exposed skin, and vesicles and bullae may occur in more sensitized individuals. (2) Common agents are listed in Table 4. (12)(13)(15)(16) Some medications, including nonsteroidal anti-inflammatory drugs, may cause both phototoxity and photoallergy.

Porphyrias are caused by the abnormal activity of enzymes involved in heme synthesis, resulting in the accumulation of various intermediates in the heme biosynthetic pathway. (17) Erythropoietic protoporphyria, the most common porphyria in children, presents with a burning, stinging, or pruritic sensation within 30 minutes of sun exposure. (18) Erythema or edema of the skin may occur with prolonged sun exposure. (17) Erythropoietic protoporphyria should be considered in infants who cry after brief exposure to sunlight. Other cutaneous porphyrias commonly develop blistering with scarring and are included in Table 2. (17)

The Condition

The patient's lesions clinically resembled lichen nitidus (LN), but this condition is not associated with sun exposure. (19) After ruling out common photodermatoses based on medical history, medication and chemical exposure, lesion morphology, and time to onset of cutaneous findings, our patient was diagnosed as having actinic LN (ALN). ALN is a recurring, seasonal variant of LN most

Table 3. Common Causes of Phototoxic Reactions (12)(13)

SYSTEMIC	TOPICAL
• Diuretics (hydrochlorothiazide, furosemide, indapamide, triamterene)	• Coal tar
• Antihypertensives (amlodipine, nifedipine)	• Benzoyl perozide
• Antiarrhythmics (amiodarone, dronedarone)	• Benzocaine
• NSAIDs (naproxen, ibuprofen, benoxaprofen, ketoprofen, celecoxib)	• Furocoumarins (commonly in oranges, lemons, limes, grapefruit, carrots, celery, parsley, and parsnips)
• Tetracyclines (doxycycline, minocycline, tetracycline)	
• Fluoroquinolones (nalidixic acid, lomefloxacin, sparfloxacin, clinafloxacin, ciprofloxacin, levofloxacin, ofloxacin, moxofloxacin	
• Sulfonamide derivatives (cotrimoxazole, dapsone, sulfasalazine)	
• Antifungals (voriconazole, itraconazole, ketoconazole, griseofulvin, fluconazole)	
• Antituberculosis (isoniazid, pyrazinamide)	
• Antimalarial (quinine, quinidine)	
• Phenothiazines (chlorpromazine, thoridazine, fluphenazine, perphenazine)	
• Alprazolam	
• Antiarrhythmics (amiodarone)	
• Atorvastatin	
• Systemic retinoids	
• Antiretrovirals (efavirenz)	

Table 4. Common Causes of Photoallergic Contact Dermatitis (12)(13)(15)(16)

SYSTEMIC	TOPICAL
• Chemotherapeutic agents (vandetanib, vemurafenib, imatinib, vinblastine) • NSAIDs (ketoprofen, piroxicam, celecoxib) • Phenothiazines (chlorpromazine, thoridazine, fluphenazine, perphenazine) • Antimalarials (quinine, quinidine) • Antiretrovirals (efavirenz) • Antiarrhythmics (amiodarone, dronedarone) • Fluoroquinolones (norfloxacin, lomefloxacin, enoxacin) • Simvastatin • Fenofibrate • Antihypertensives (hydrochlorothiazide, captopril, ramipril, enalapril, valsartan) • Chlordiazepoxide	• NSAIDs (ketoprofen, diclofenac, benzydamine) • Acyclovir • Dibucaine injection • Hydrocortisone • Suncreens (containing p-aminobenzoid acid, benzophenones, cinnamates, salicylates, octocrylene, oxybenzone) • Chlorpromazine gel • Chlorhexidine • Hexachlorophene • Bithionol • Fragrances (containing 6-methylcoumarin, musk ambrette, sandalwood oil)

NSAID=nonsteroidal anti-inflammatory drug.

frequently occurring in pediatric or young adult patients with darker complexions (Fitzpatrick skin types IV–VI) after sun exposure. (20) Although rare, ALN is likely underrecognized. (21)

Classic LN occurs primarily in school-age children and demonstrates numerous, discrete, asymptomatic, monomorphic, pinhead-sized, skin-colored to hypopigmented papules clustered in groups on both sun-exposed and sun-protected skin. (19)(20) LN follows a chronic course and resolves over several months to years, after which recurrence is uncommon. (19)(21) Koebnerization of lesions (the development of skin lesions at sites of trauma) is a useful clue to aid in diagnosis of LN and often results from scratching. Despite morphologically similar lesions, ALN can be differentiated from the classic form of LN by its timing, seasonal recurrence, and photodistribution. Typically, ALN appears 24 to 48 hours after sun exposure on the uncovered skin while sparing skin protected from sunlight. (20) Histologic analyses of LN and ALN reveal a ball-shaped lichenoid infiltrate of lymphocytes, histiocytes, plasma cells, and rare giant cells in the papillary dermis with epidermal thinning and downward extension of rete ridges at the lateral margins of the infiltrate described as a "ball-in-claw." (20)(21)(22)(23)(24)(25)(26)(27)(28)(29)

The diagnosis of ALN can be made clinically, and our patient's history and physical examination were characteristic. A skin biopsy was discussed with the patient's father, but given the high clinical suspicion for ALN, the biopsy

was deferred. Skin lesions often resolve over several weeks with photoprotection alone, although topical corticosteroids may be used for symptomatic relief of itching. (22) Sun protection is critical in preventing future recurrences.

Lessons for the Clinician

- Actinic lichen nitidus (ALN) is considered a rare condition that is more common in patients with skin of color, although it is likely underdiagnosed in patients of all skin types.
- Recognition of ALN's characteristic features may expedite diagnosis and avoid invasive procedures.
- Sun protection with sunscreen or clothing is important in limiting the recurrence of ALN.
- When evaluating cutaneous concerns, placing the patient in a gown may aid in identification of the sun-exposed skin distribution.
- Although the differential diagnosis for photosensitivity disorders is broad, careful evaluation of the clinical history, timing of the onset and resolution of lesions, associated symptoms, medication or other exposures, and lesion morphology can help narrow the differential diagnosis.

References for this article can be found at
https://doi.org/10.1542/pir.2021-005359.

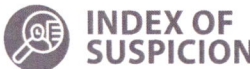
INDEX OF SUSPICION

Multiple Hyperpigmented Lesions in a Young Girl

Katie Dreher, BS,* Jonathan W. Rick, MD,† Hugh Nymeyer, MD, PhD,† Megan S. Evans, MD†

*College of Medicine, University of Arkansas for Medical Sciences, Little Rock, AR
†Department of Dermatology, University of Arkansas for Medical Sciences, Little Rock, AR

PRESENTATION

An 18-month-old, otherwise healthy girl presents to the pediatric dermatology clinic for the evaluation of numerous hyperpigmented spots on her skin. The spots started on her middle back around age 2 months and gradually spread to involve most of her trunk, neck, and proximal extremities. She was previously referred by her primary care physician to the genetics clinic due to concern for multiple café-au-lait macules (CALMs). To rule out neurofibromatosis type 1 (NF1), Legius syndrome, and related conditions, an 18-gene panel was run for *NF1, SPRED1,* and other RASopathy-associated genes. Results of the genetic testing were normal.

The patient has been growing well and meeting all appropriate developmental milestones. Review of systems is negative for fever, flushing, and syncope but positive for several recent episodes of diarrhea. On physical examination there are numerous well-circumscribed, hyperpigmented macules, papules, and patches present diffusely across the back, abdomen, neck, and extremities of the patient. There is no evidence of axillary or inguinal freckling, hepatomegaly, splenomegaly, or lymphadenopathy. Shortly after rubbing one of the hyperpigmented macules firmly with a tongue depressor, the lesion becomes erythematous and raised. On further questioning, the patient's mother reports that the lesions do occasionally become similarly red and elevated, possibly in association with environmental temperature changes.

DISCUSSION

Differential Diagnosis
The differential diagnosis for our patient's presentation included cutaneous mastocytosis, CALMs (idiopathic or related to a syndrome such as NF1 or Legius syndrome), urticaria, and melanocytic nevi.

Actual Diagnosis
Maculopapular cutaneous mastocytosis (MPCM).

The Condition
MPCM, previously called urticaria pigmentosa, is the most common type of mastocytosis seen in the pediatric population. (1) The cutaneous mastocytoses are characterized by mast cell proliferation in the skin, with symptoms caused by release of mast cell mediators, including tryptase, histamine, leukotrienes, and prostaglandins. (2)(3)(4) The cause of this proliferation is poorly understood,

AUTHOR DISCLOSURE: Ms Dreher and Drs Rick, Nymeyer, and Evans have disclosed no financial relationships relevant to this article. This commentary does not contain a discussion of an unapproved/investigative use of a commercial product/device.

but mutations in c-KIT, a type of receptor tyrosine kinase, have been implicated. (5) Development of the disease is typically sporadic rather than inherited, and up to two-thirds of cases present in infancy or childhood. (5)(6)

Childhood-onset MPCM typically presents as tan-to-brown, polymorphic patches and plaques (Fig 1); round, monomorphic macules and papules may also be seen. (6)(7) The lesions favor the trunk and classically spare the face, palms, and soles. (6)(7) Typically, lesions appear within the first year of life. (3)(6) They periodically become erythematous, swollen, and pruritic in association with a variety of triggers, and subsequent blistering may also occur in children younger than 2 years. (3)(5) Triggers include exposures known to induce mast cell degranulation, including extreme hot and cold environmental temperatures, fever, rapid changes in patient temperature, rubbing of lesions, snake and Hymenoptera venom, infections, surgeries, emotional stress, and sleep deprivation. (3)(8) Drugs, including aspirin, nonsteroidal anti-inflammatories, narcotics, dextromethorphan, anticholinergics, magnetic resonance imaging contrast media, and some systemic anesthetic drugs may also result in flares. (3) Patients with MPCM may develop systemic symptoms related to mast cell degranulation, including flushing, dizziness, and headaches. (1)(5)(8) Gastrointestinal symptoms, such as abdominal pain, diarrhea, nausea, and vomiting, are the most common extracutaneous symptoms and are found in 40% of these children. (1)(4)(8) Due to an increase in mast cells, the primary cell type implicated in anaphylaxis, children with MPCM are at slightly higher risk for anaphylaxis than the general pediatric population. (9) These reactions can be IgE-mediated or due to nonspecific activation of these clonal, hyperresponsive mast cells. (9) Although this type of response is rare and often without an identified cause, patients should exhibit caution by avoiding the previously mentioned triggers whenever possible. (9) Interestingly, patients with mastocytosis have been found to be at higher risk for both more frequent and more severe anaphylactic reactions to Hymenoptera venom, and patients should be made aware of this risk. (10)

Diagnosis of MPCM is typically clinical and is strongly suggested by a positive Darier sign on physical examination. (4) The Darier sign occurs when a lesion is firmly rubbed with a blunt tool, resulting in degranulation of mast cells and development of erythema, swelling, and pruritus within several minutes (Fig 2). (5)(7) The test should also be performed on a nearby unaffected area of skin and is considered positive if it occurs only over the lesion. (5) Often, this sign alone is sufficient for diagnosis. If the diagnosis is uncertain, a biopsy can be performed, showing increased mast cells in the dermal papillae and surrounding superficial vasculature. (3) Stains such as

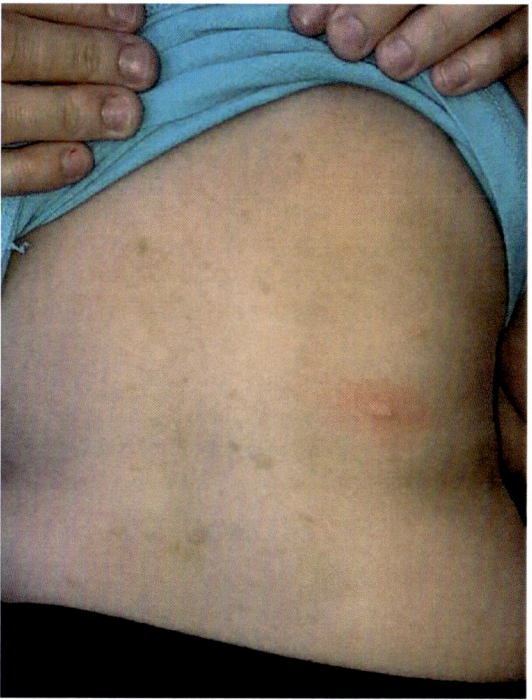

Figure 1. Multiple tan macules, papules, and patches on the trunk of an infant with maculopapular cutaneous mastocytosis.

Figure 2. Erythema and edema resulting from rubbing of a lesion of cutaneous mastocytosis, demonstrating a positive Darier sign.

Giemsa and toluidine blue, as well as immunohistochemical stains targeting CD117 and tryptase, can assist in identifying mast cells. (2)(3)(8)

The tan-to-brown coloration of MPCM lesions may be confused with that of CALMs, raising suspicion for syndromic conditions associated with multiple CALMs, such as NF1. (11) The Darier sign, as described previously herein, is an easy-to-perform bedside test that can differentiate MPCM from the multiple CALMs seen in NF1 and related disorders. In addition, borders of lesions of cutaneous mastocytosis tend to be less well-defined than those of CALMs. History gathering can also be helpful; the family may report periodic episodes of redness and swelling of the lesions, which would not be an expected observation in the case of CALMs. In addition to MPCM, other less common forms of cutaneous mastocytosis may present in children. Mastocytomas are differentiated from MPCM by the presence of 3 or fewer lesions. (7) Diffuse cutaneous mastocytosis is characterized by generalized skin involvement, resulting in diffusely erythematous, thickened skin with the tendency to blister. (7) Other conditions that may be confused with MPCM include urticaria, in which individual lesions typically last for only hours and lack the hyperpigmentation found in MPCM, as well as melanocytic nevi, which do not exhibit the Darier sign. (12)

Management

The management of MPCM in children is focused on symptom control and flare avoidance. (13) Many patients do not require treatment, but all families should be counseled about avoidance of common triggers of mast cell degranulation. (2)(5)(8) In patients whose lesions are primarily of cosmetic concern, topical corticosteroids under occlusion can be considered. (2) For patients whose lesions are symptomatic, scheduled or as-needed H_1 antihistamines are first-line therapy. (2)(13) H_2 antihistamines and cromolyn sodium can be added if symptoms are poorly controlled and may be especially beneficial in patients experiencing chronic gastrointestinal symptoms. (2)(3)(5)(13) Although controversial, provision of autoinjectable epinephrine to patients with extensive skin involvement, significant systemic symptoms, or high levels of serum tryptase may be considered due to the increased risk of anaphylactic reactions in these children, although use of these injectors is infrequent. (9)(14)(15) These prescriptions are especially recommended in patients with a personal history of anaphylaxis. (15)

Systemic mastocytosis is rare in children, and extensive diagnostic studies to rule out this condition should be avoided in typical cases of cutaneous mastocytosis. (2)(5) Systemic mastocytosis is defined by mast cell accumulation in at least 1 organ besides the skin. (3) Commonly affected organs include the bones, spleen, liver, and lymph nodes, which may lead to skeletal lesions, demineralization, and bone pain, as well as hepatosplenomegaly and lymphadenopathy. (3) The presence of the extracutaneous symptoms previously mentioned are not predictive of systemic involvement, but an increase in their severity or the presence of bone pain, hypotension, or syncope is concerning for rising mast cell mediators seen in association with systemic mastocytosis. (3)(5) A thorough history and physical examination should be performed to investigate for these findings. A complete blood cell count with differential count, tryptase level, and liver function studies are also reasonable initial diagnostic tests, although some clinicians may choose to omit these studies in patients with limited skin involvement and no systemic symptoms. (2)(5) Persistently elevated or increasing levels of tryptase, cytopenias, or abnormal liver function studies raise concern for extracutaneous involvement; a bone marrow biopsy and more frequent clinical monitoring may be indicated in these patients. (2)(8)

Prognosis

The overall prognosis for childhood-onset MPCM is excellent, and studies have shown little overall effect on quality of life in these patients. (1) In many children, complete resolution occurs before puberty, and continued improvement is typically seen in those whose disease persists. (1)(2)(6)

Patient Course

Laboratory evaluation consisting of a complete blood cell count, tryptase level, and liver function studies were obtained, all yielding normal results. The patient's mother was counseled on avoidance of triggers and use of diphenhydramine as needed for flares. The patient was prescribed an epinephrine autoinjector due to her increased risk of anaphylaxis. On follow-up 3 months later, she was experiencing fewer flares of her lesions, and the previous episodes of diarrhea had resolved. The natural history of the disease and likelihood of resolution with age was reviewed. The patient was instructed to follow up yearly.

Lessons for the Clinician

1. Maculopapular cutaneous mastocytosis (MPCM) is the most common form of mastocytosis in children. (1) Its lesions may be mistaken for café-au-lait macules (CALMs), melanocytic nevi, or urticaria.

2. The Darier sign is a simple bedside test that can be performed by pediatricians to help distinguish lesions of cutaneous mastocytosis from CALMs. This test may help avoid expensive genetic evaluation for conditions associated with multiple CALMs, such as neurofibromatosis type 1. (5)(7)

3. Management of MPCM in children includes trigger avoidance and symptomatic treatment with H_1 antihistamines with or without H_2 antihistamines and cromolyn sodium. (2)(3)(13)

4. Anaphylaxis is seen in higher rates in children with extensive skin involvement, high tryptase levels, and significant systemic symptoms. Prescribing autoinjectable epinephrine should be considered in these patients. (9)(15)

5. A thorough history and physical examination with limited laboratory tests, including a complete blood cell count, serum tryptase level, and liver function studies, are reasonable initial tests to rule out systemic mastocytosis due to its rarity in children. (5)

References for this article can be found at
https://doi.org/10.1542/pir.2021-005106.

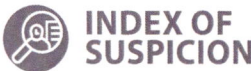

INDEX OF
SUSPICION

Fever and Perianal Erythema in a 5-year-old Boy

Fatima Abdo, MD,* Deborah Tyokighir, MD,* Yojana Sunkoj, MD,* Robert R. Wittler, MD*

*Kansas University School of Medicine–Wichita, Wichita, KS

CASE PRESENTATION

A 5-year-old boy with pre–B-cell acute lymphocytic leukemia presents with fever, nausea, vomiting, and decreased oral intake during the past 24 hours. He had a temperature of 102°F (38.9°C) at home and was brought to the hospital due to concern for chemotherapy-induced neutropenia with fever. He had a history of constipation with painful bowel movements and a history of recurrent perianal erythema. At home he takes lactulose, oxycodone, ondansetron, and diphenhydramine as needed along with his chemotherapy regimen. He was last hospitalized 2 weeks earlier for fever and neutropenia and received empirical intravenous (IV) cefepime. At that hospitalization he was noted to have perianal erythema, and a swab of the perianal area was obtained and ordered as a culture for group A streptococcus (GAS). The antigen was negative for GAS, and no GAS was isolated on the culture. A blood culture from that admission was negative. He clinically improved and was discharged after 48 hours without further antibiotic therapy.

Physical examination was remarkable for circumferential perianal erythema with a sharp border. A perianal fissure was not noted. A perianal swab was sent for culture. Blood work was remarkable for complete blood cell count (reference values): white blood cell count, 300/μL (0.3×10⁹/L) (500–1,500/μL [0.5–1.5×10⁹/L]); hemoglobin level, 9.8 g/dL (98 g/L) (11.5–14.5 g/dL [115–145 g/L]); hematocrit level, 27.0% (35%–43%); platelet count, 5,000×10³/μL (5,000×10⁹/L) (150–400,000×10³/μL [150–400,000×10⁹/L]); and absolute neutrophil count, 100/μL (0.1×10⁹/L) (2,000–9,000/μL [2.0–9.0×10⁹/L]). He was admitted to the hospital and started on IV cefepime for fever and neutropenia.

The blood culture obtained from the port-a-cath on admission was initially reported as gram-positive cocci resembling streptococcus. The swab obtained from the perianal area had heavy growth of β-hemolytic colonies. Latex agglutination for GAS was negative.

DISCUSSION

Differential Diagnosis

This patient's history of leukemia and presentation with fever and neutropenia complicated the evaluation due to the concern for possible invasive or opportunistic infection in addition to the perianal dermatitis. The differential diagnosis for perianal dermatitis includes infectious and noninfectious conditions such as candidiasis, *Staphylococcus aureus* infection, irritant dermatitis, eczema, psoriasis, seborrheic dermatitis, trauma, and sexual abuse. (1)(2) There was no history of eczema, psoriasis, seborrheic dermatitis, trauma, or irritant exposure. Sexual

Author Disclosure: Drs Abdo, Tyokighir, Sunkoj, and Wittler have disclosed no financial relationships relevant to this article. This commentary does contain a brief discussion of the use of streptococcal antigen assays that have been used by clinicians in the diagnosis of perianal dermatitis but are indicated only for pharyngeal swabs. The commentary notes that those antigen assays are indicated only for pharyngeal specimens and will detect only group A streptococcus and not groups B, C, or G β-hemolytic streptococci.

abuse was not suspected. The physical examination findings were not consistent with *Candida* infection because there was no scaling or papulovesicular lesions and it did not extend to other areas of the perineum. There were no pustules or papules suggestive of *S aureus* infection. The physical examination noting a sharp border of erythema along with a previous episode made perianal dermatitis due to β-hemolytic streptococci the most likely etiology.

Actual Diagnosis and Patient Course

The blood culture organism was identified as group C streptococcus (GCS). With the perianal swab from the previous admission being negative for GAS, specific testing for GCS on the perianal swab was requested and was positive in this case. Repeated blood cultures obtained from the port-a-cath on hospital days 2, 3, and 4 had no growth. It was concluded that the primary focus of infection was the GCS perianal dermatitis with secondary bacteremia and not a catheter-associated bloodstream infection. With resolution of his fever and neutropenia he was discharged to complete a 10-day course of IV ceftriaxone through the port-a-cath from the first negative blood culture, and he did well. He has not had a recurrence of perianal dermatitis.

The Condition

β-Hemolytic GCS and group G streptococcus (GGS) causing human infections taxonomically are a single subspecies, *Streptococcus dysgalactiae* subsp *equisimilis*. (3)(4) GCS and GGS can cause diseases similar to GAS, with infection of the skin, soft tissue, and respiratory tract; pharyngitis; bacteremia; and endocarditis. (3)(4) A retrospective study from 1999 to 2013 in Norway noted a significant increase in the incidence of GCS and GGS invasive infections. (4)

GAS is the predominant cause of perianal infectious dermatitis in children. (1)(2)(5) β-Hemolytic group B streptococcus (GBS) has been noted to be the most common etiology of perianal cellulitis in adults. (6) A case series of children from New York City, however, noted a predominance of *S aureus* as the etiology for perianal bacterial dermatitis. (7) The presence of papules and pustules and the extension of erythema onto the buttocks generally accompany *S aureus* infection in contrast to GAS perianal dermatitis. GCS and GGS have been infrequently reported as causal organisms for perianal dermatitis. (1)(2)(5)

It is not unusual for the diagnosis of perianal infectious dermatitis to be missed for a prolonged period. (2)(8)(9) The symptoms of perianal infectious dermatitis (eg, perianal itching) are similar to those of various other conditions, although the physical examination is fairly specific

for streptococcal infection, which Serban (2) described as "sharply demarcated perianal circumferential edematous erythema extending 2-4 cm around the anus, sometimes with white exudate, pseudomembranes, and superficial anal fissures or cracks." Perianal infectious dermatitis occurs predominantly in children between ages 6 months and 10 years. (2) The maximum incidence is between 3 and 6 years of age. (2) The diagnosis is confirmed with culture. It is important that the microbiology laboratory understand that β-hemolytic streptococci other than GAS are being considered with perianal dermatitis. With throat cultures, microbiology laboratories may report growth of GAS only because isolation of GCS and GGS is of uncertain clinical significance because they often colonize the pharynx, and they are not known to result in acute rheumatic fever. Streptococcal antigen tests for GAS have been used for the diagnosis of streptococcal perianal dermatitis, (8) but they are approved only for pharyngeal specimens. Rapid streptococcal antigen tests will not detect GBS, GCS, or GGS infection. (10)

Treatment

β-Hemolytic streptococci, including GCS and GGS, are susceptible to penicillins and other β-lactam drugs. Oral penicillin, amoxicillin, or cephalexin for 7 to 10 days is commonly used for treatment of infectious perianal dermatitis. Topical mupiricin in addition to an oral antibiotic may have added benefit. (2) Relapses after treatment are common. (2)(8)(9) Patients with bacteremia from β-hemolytic streptococci are treated for 10 to 14 days.

Lessons for the Clinician

- A demarcated perianal circumferential edematous erythema is characteristic of streptococcal perianal dermatitis.
- Group A streptococcus is the most frequent etiology for perianal infectious dermatitis, and other β-hemolytic streptococci (groups B, C, G) are also causative agents with a clinically indistinguishable presentation.
- The presence of papules and pustules would be consistent with *Staphylococcus aureus* perianal dermatitis.
- Culture confirms the diagnosis of infectious perianal dermatitis. Rapid streptococcal antigen tests may aid in diagnosing group A streptococcus, but they are approved only for pharyngeal specimens. They will be negative for other β-hemolytic streptococci.

References for this article can be found at
https://doi.org/10.1542/pir.2021-005138.

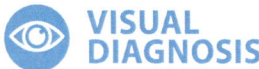
VISUAL DIAGNOSIS

Salt Treatment for a Lesion with Recurrent Bleeding in an 11-year-old Child

Ahmet Miguel Yildirim, MD,* Jeffrey Lancaster, MD,[†] Zachary Zinn, MD*

*Department of Dermatology and [†]Department of Pediatrics-Division of Pediatric Hospital Medicine, West Virginia University, Morgantown, WV

PRESENTATION

An 11-year-old previously healthy girl presents to the clinic with a lesion over her right thumb. Four weeks before presentation the patient received a splinter in her right thumb from the wood flooring of her back deck that was immediately removed with her fingernails. No additional wound care was required at that time. A raised lesion appeared 4 days after splinter removal. During the ensuing 4 weeks, the lesion enlarged and bled repetitively. She bandaged the lesion daily and washed her finger with regular soap and water. Our patient is right-handed, and function of her hand is not impaired. She has not sought medical advice elsewhere. The mother notes no associated fever or other lesions present. There are no recent sick contacts or travel history. All immunizations are up to date, including influenza. She did not receive the COVID-19 vaccine. Except for a daily multivitamin, there is no medication use. The patient has not begun menstruating. Family history is negative for bleeding disorders or skin cancers. There is no history of similar lesions.

On physical examination the patient appears well. BMI is at the 40th percentile. Physical examination reveals an erythematous, friable, vascularized papule measuring 5×5 mm on the right distal thumb (Fig 1). Both hands are fully mobile with 5/5 strength and intact sensation throughout. The remaining cutaneous and mucus membrane examination findings are normal. Laboratory tests and imaging are not ordered.

The patient is instructed to treat the lesion by applying soft paraffin around the periphery of the lesion and then covering the lesion with table salt followed by occlusion. The family notes that bleeding immediately ceased on salt application. One day after initiation of treatment the lesion is markedly less erythematous, is dry, and appears pedunculated (Fig 2). Clinical examination findings and response to treatment confirm the diagnosis.

DIAGNOSIS

The differential diagnosis included pyogenic granuloma, Spitz nevus, amelanotic melanoma, and bacillary angiomatosis. This lesion appeared to be most consistent with pyogenic granuloma. This is a benign vascular growth that normally presents as a friable, vascularized papule or polyp of the skin and mucous membranes after minor injuries or changes in hormone levels. Commonly, it can present on the finger, lip, face, or tongue and will typically bleed.

Dr Yildirim's current affiliation is Inova Health Systems, Falls Church, VA.

AUTHOR DISCLOSURE: Mr Yildirim and Drs Lancaster and Zinn have disclosed no financial relationships relevant to this article. This commentary does not contain a discussion of an unapproved/ investigative use of commercial product/ device.

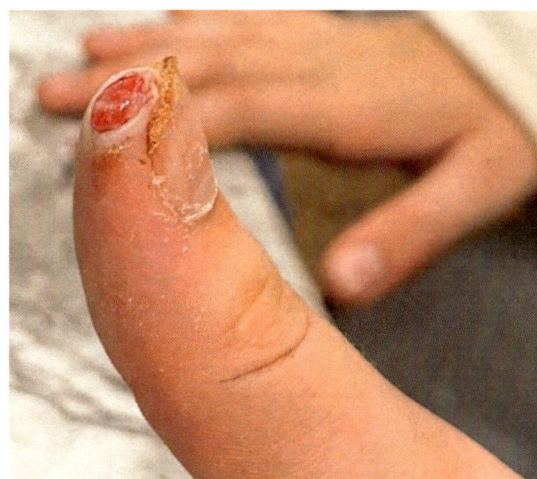

Figure 1. Lesion at presentation is a vascularized papule measuring 5 × 5 mm on the right distal thumb.

DISCUSSION

Pyogenic granuloma represents 0.5% of all skin nodules in children, with the oral variant occurring in approximately 5% of pregnancies. (1)(2) It is more frequently seen in children and young adults, with frequency declining with increased age. It affects males more often than females; however, the oral variant is 2 times more common in females, likely due to hormonal changes during pregnancy, and typically presents on the gingiva. (3) In addition, pyogenic granulomas have been associated with retinoid therapy in patients treated for acne and psoriasis. (4) Lesions resulting from pregnancy and medication use typically resolve after parturition and withdrawal of the causative

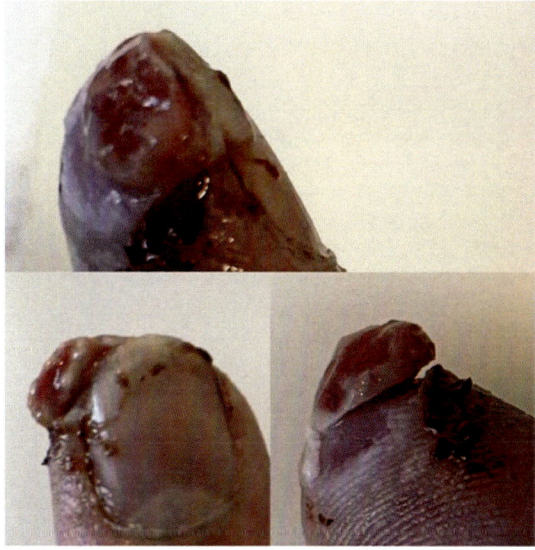

Figure 2. The lesion appears less erythematous and pedunculated after 1 day of topical salt application.

agent, respectively. However, for refractory pyogenic granulomas, treatment may be warranted to reduce bleeding.

As an acquired vascular tumor of the skin, pyogenic granulomas present as an outpouching of granulation tissue in early stages with an edematous stroma that contains an aggregate of inflammatory infiltrate. In later stages, small pyogenic granulomas may regress to form scar tissue. (4) Histopathologically, pyogenic granulomas appear as lobular growths in the endothelial-lined lumen of capillaries and venules. (5)

Current treatment modalities include topical therapies (imiquimod, timolol + trichloroacetic acid, propranolol, ingenol mebutate), intralesional injection (triamcinolone acetonide, bleomycin), intralesional sclerotherapy (monoethanolamine oleate), cryotherapy (nitrous oxide, liquid nitrogen), curettage, electrodessication, systemic therapies (prednisone ± levofloxacin hydrate), surgical excision, and laser therapy. (6) Surgical excision is the most performed treatment. Recurrence of pyogenic granuloma after treatment has been reported. The recurrence rate varies from 2.94% to 43.5% for surgical excision to 1.62% for cryotherapy. (1)(7) The recurrence rates for less commonly performed treatment modalities are not available.

Recently, the novel application of topical salt has been described as a promising treatment for pyogenic granulomas. Deriving inspiration from 2 previous cases, which used common table salt to completely resolve umbilical granulomas, Daruwalla and Dhurat (8) used salt on 5 patients with known pyogenic granuloma. They applied commercial salt over the entire lesion, protecting the surrounding skin with paraffin, and occluded the area with adhesive surgical tape. Depending on the size of the initial lesion, complete resolution occurred in 7 to 14 days, with no recurrence noted at 1-month follow-up. (8)

It is believed the salt creates a hygroscopic environment under the occlusive dressing that acts as a drying agent or adsorbent. (8) Fluid shifts from the intracellular space to the hyperosmolar extracellular space, causing cell size to decrease and disruption of blood supply. Over time, cellular necrosis leads to resolution of the lesion.

To confirm initial findings, Daruwalla et al (9) performed a prospective open-label study of 50 individuals with pyogenic granuloma. All the patients were treated with topical salt and followed up for complications and recurrence. The authors found that 100% of the patients had complete resolution of their lesion without residual scarring, and 94% witnessed a decrease in bleeding from the lesion almost immediately after intervention. The mean time to complete resolution was 15 days. Of note, this study did not include refractory pyogenic granuloma as an inclusion criterion, and, consequently, the population may have had a low risk of recurrence. Another case report suggests that salt may also be effective in a recurrent oral lesion, specifically, overlying the right half of the lower lip, after previous partial excision. After a failed shave excision, electrocautery, and application of silver nitrate, and multiple cycles of cryotherapy, an at-home administration of salt with petroleum jelly on the perilesional area and overlying gauze resulted in complete resolution of the oral lesion after 2 weeks with no recurrence. (10)

Although salt is a potential treatment for pyogenic granuloma, salt application should not be used as a first-line intervention when the diagnosis is uncertain. Surgical removal is preferred for lesions with uncertain etiology to confirm the diagnosis via histopathologic analysis. One would not want to miss a diagnosis of amelanotic melanoma. Although amelanotic melanoma was considered in the differential diagnosis of this patient, the diagnosis of pyogenic granuloma was more certain given her clinical presentation and age.

Given its inexpensive cost, wide availability, and noninvasive modality, salt can be considered an option for treatment of pyogenic granulomas on both the skin and lips. Specifically, salt may be a viable alternative to more invasive therapy such as surgical excision or cryotherapy. In addition, in the largest case series to date, salt led to the resolution of pyogenic granulomas within approximately 2 weeks. Although direct comparison of pain associated with salt application versus other surgical modalities has not been performed, salt application is minimally painful, with a mild sensation of stinging during application. (10) Salt application could be a viable treatment option for pyogenic granuloma, especially in patients who want to avoid surgical excision given that the clinical diagnosis is certain.

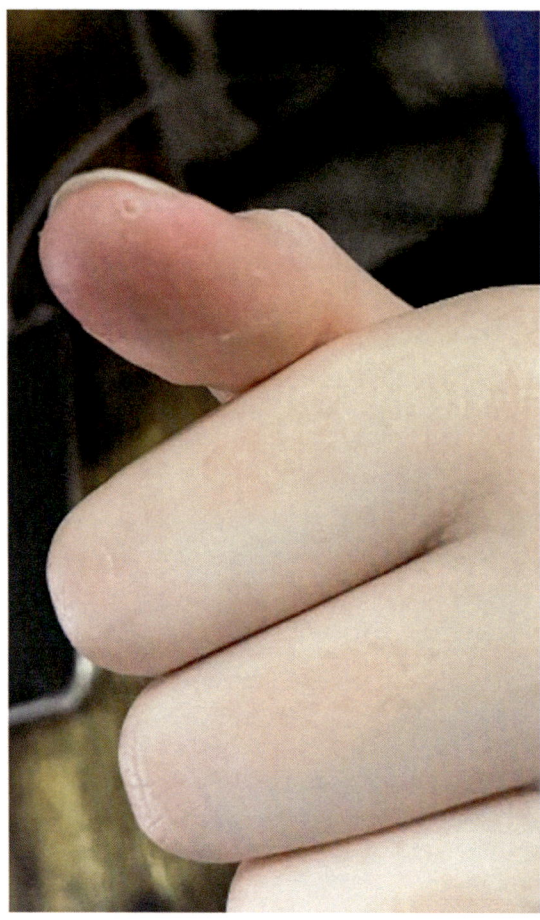

Figure 3. Complete resolution of the lesion with no scarring after 7 days of topical salt application.

PATIENT COURSE

The mother was instructed to remove the bandage and reapply the soft paraffin and salt daily until lesion resolution. The patient noted significant improvement after 2 at-home applications, with complete resolution on day 7 of daily application (Fig 3). There have been no reports of lesion recurrence 6 weeks after discontinuation of therapy. She currently has no limitations in using her thumb in her regular day-to-day activities.

Summary

- Pyogenic granuloma is a benign vascular growth that normally presents as a friable, vascularized papule or polyp of the skin and mucous membranes that recurrently bleeds.

- Current treatment modalities for pyogenic granulomas are effective, with low risk of recurrence and residual scarring; however, these treatments can often be invasive.

- In the treatment of pyogenic granulomas, table salt is inexpensive, widely available, noninvasive, and seemingly effective.

- Surgical excision and histopathologic analysis are recommended before other medical interventions to confirm the diagnosis and rule out malignancy when the clinical diagnosis is uncertain.

References for this article can be found at https://doi.org/10.1542/pir.2022-005581.

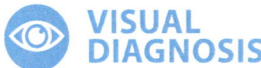
VISUAL DIAGNOSIS

Targetoid Rash in an Infant—Hit the Target!

Blake A. Boehm, BS,* Kathy Kolodziejski, DO,† Aparna Roy, MD,*† Gurinder Kumar, MD*†

*Case Western Reserve University School of Medicine, Cleveland, OH
†MetroHealth Medical Center, Cleveland, OH

PRESENTATION

A previously healthy 9-month-old boy presents to the emergency department with 2 days of a migratory urticarial rash. The rash started on the back of his neck and quickly progressed over the face, trunk, and extremities, sparing the palms of the hands and soles of the feet. According to his parents, the child's face appeared swollen since the rash started. He has mild nasal congestion but does not have any respiratory issues, feeding difficulties, or change in bowel or bladder habits. Eight days ago, the child had a fever, congestion, and cough and was diagnosed as having acute otitis media. He was started on amoxicillin, and his symptoms improved until 2 days ago when the rash appeared. The last dose of amoxicillin was 2 days ago. The boy's parents report that the child had taken amoxicillin twice in the past and developed a rash (without fever) on 1 of these occasions. The previous rash was a maculopapular rash over the trunk but not like the current one.

The boy has rice and oat intolerance but no known allergies. His family history is remarkable for a cousin who also developed a rash in the setting of amoxicillin use, a father with a childhood history of asthma, and a paternal aunt with lupus. The patient is not currently taking any medications, nor has he used any new soaps, detergents, or topical creams. There is no history of international travel. He has had no known sick contacts, although he is in day care. He is up to date on his immunizations and last received a vaccination 10 weeks ago.

Vital signs in the emergency department are as follows: temperature, 101.3°F (38.5°C); heart rate, 156 beats/min; respiratory rate, 24 breaths/min; and oxygen saturation, 98% on room air. Physical examination is notable for a diffuse rash over the head, chest, back, and extremities, sparing the palms and the soles of the feet (Fig 1). The rash is worse in the axilla and groin. Individual lesions are raised and annular, with a dusky center and erythematous border. There is no sloughing of the skin, bullae, vesicles, or oral mucosal involvement. Dermographism was noted. Cardiac examination findings are normal without murmur, lungs are clear to auscultation, and abdomen is soft, nontender, and nondistended, with no hepatosplenomegaly. There is no lymphadenopathy.

Laboratory evaluation demonstrates mild anemia (hemoglobin level, 11.0 g/dL [110 g/L]; hematocrit value, 32.2%), thrombocytosis (platelet count, $428 \times 10^3/\mu L$ [$428 \times 10^9/L$]), and a normal white blood cell count (14,000/μL [$14.0 \times 10^9/L$]). Findings from the basic metabolic panel, hepatic function panel, and urinalysis are within normal limits. The C-reactive protein level is within normal limits. The respiratory virus panel is positive for rhinovirus and negative for COVID-19,

AUTHOR DISCLOSURE: Mr Boehm and Drs Kolodziejski, Roy, and Kumar have disclosed no financial relationships relevant to this article. This commentary does not contain a discussion of an unapproved/investigative use of a commercial product/device.

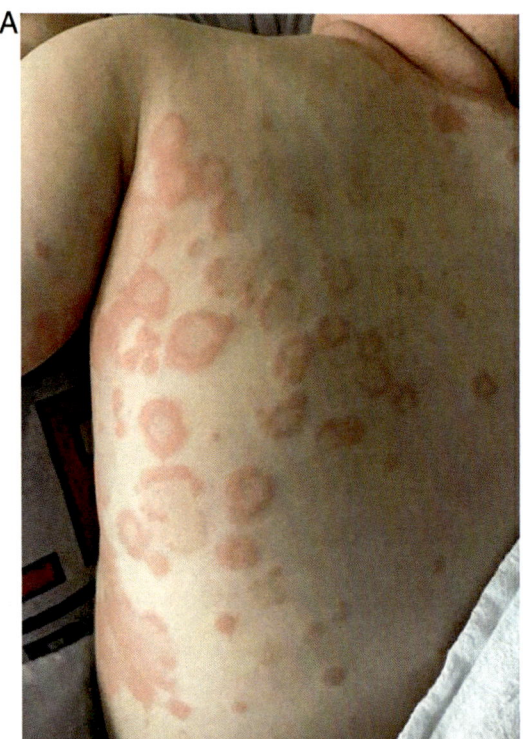

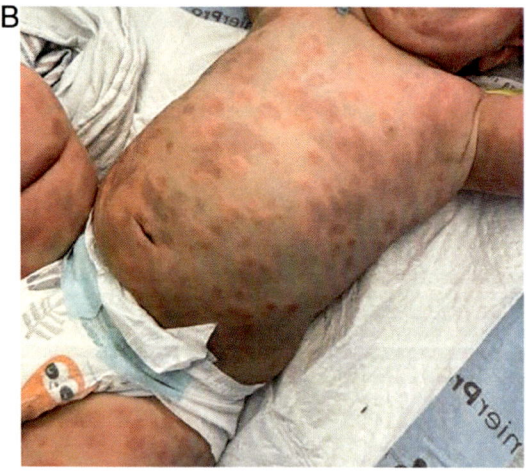

Figure 1. Rash over the patient's back (A) and chest and abdomen (B) on admission. The lesions are annular and raised and have a central clearing or dusky appearance with an erythematous border.

influenza, respiratory syncytial virus, parainfluenza virus, metapneumovirus, adenovirus, bocavirus, *Chlamydophila pneumoniae,* and *Mycoplasma pneumoniae.* Herpes simplex virus (HSV1, HSV2) DNA polymerase chain reaction is also negative. Chest radiography is notable for perihilar bronchovascular thickening. Blood culture is sent to the laboratory and remained sterile. The clinical course confirmed the diagnosis.

DIAGNOSIS

Erythema multiforme, urticaria multiforme, and serum sickness–like reaction were at the top of the differential diagnosis. Acute urticaria, erythema chronicum migrans, autoinflammatory disorder, acute hemorrhagic edema of infancy, urticarial vasculitis, viral exanthems, and serum sickness were also considered although less likely. Based on the clinical course and the patient's exposures, urticaria multiforme was the most likely diagnosis.

DISCUSSION

Urticaria multiforme is a common, although often misdiagnosed, dermatologic condition of the pediatric population characterized by large, annular, polycyclic wheals that may have a dusky center or central clearing. (1)(2) It is a subtype of acute urticaria and was first termed *acute annular urticaria* by Tamayo-Sanchez et al (2) in 1997, and later referred to as *urticaria multiforme* by Shah et al (1) in 2007. Urticaria multiforme primarily affects young children 4 months to 4 years of age. (2) Individual lesions typically resolve within 24 hours; however, the rash may persist for up to 12 days. In addition to the rash, patients may experience low-grade fever, pruritus, dermographism, and edema of the face, hands, and feet. (1)(3) Dermographism is transient mast cell–mediated erythema and swelling of the skin in response to mechanical irritation (eg, itching, rubbing). (4) Urticaria multiforme is believed to be a histamine-mediated hypersensitivity reaction to a medication or infection, typically viral or bacterial. It may be either IgE dependent or independent. (1)(5) When a particular medication is suspected to have induced a patient's urticaria multiforme, it is reasonable to recommend future avoidance of this medication if possible.

Although the exact etiology of urticaria multiforme is not yet completely understood, many children have a preceding infection, immunization, or medication use. Upper respiratory tract infections, otitis media, and symptoms consistent with viral illness have been observed in many of these children, although the causative organism is often not identified. Medications commonly associated with urticaria multiforme include antibiotics such as amoxicillin, macrolides, furazolidone, and cephalosporins, as well as antipyretics, including aspirin and acetaminophen. (1)(2)(3)(6) At times it may be challenging to determine whether the trigger was a medication or the disease for which the medication was used.

Urticaria multiforme can be diagnosed based on history and clinical presentation, without the need for biopsy of the lesion or extensive diagnostic evaluation. Two dermatologic

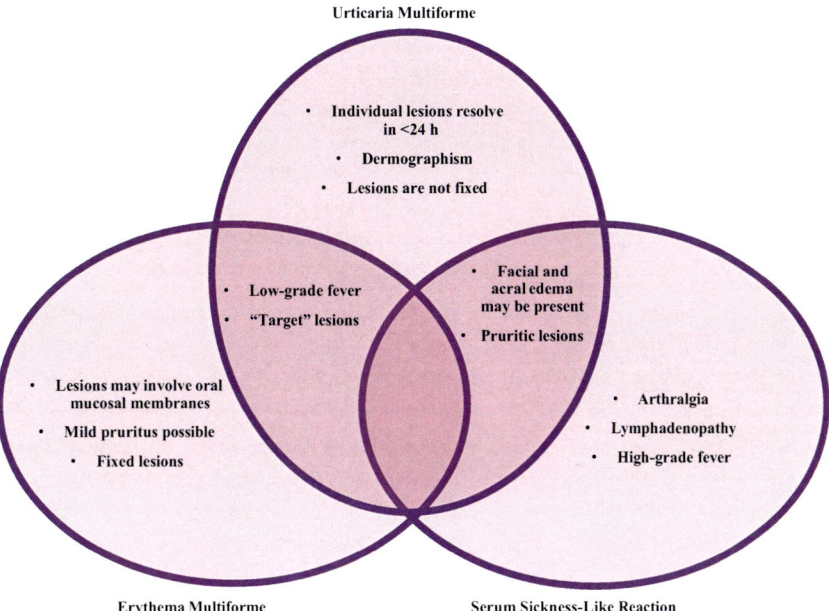

Figure 2. Diagram comparing the clinical features of urticaria multiforme, erythema multiforme, and serum sickness–like reaction. Although the rashes in these conditions may appear similar on cursory inspection, key features can help distinguish these conditions.

conditions that may be confused with urticaria multiforme are erythema multiforme and serum sickness–like reaction. Figure 2 compares important clinical features of each condition. Erythema multiforme is an immune-mediated dermatologic condition that can develop in response to infection, medication use, and immunization, as well as other triggers. (7) Infection is the primary cause of erythema multiforme, with herpes simplex virus being a common trigger. Erythema multiforme is characterized by target lesions consisting of a central area of epidermal necrosis that may blister and 3 surrounding concentric rings: an inner erythematous ring; a middle edematous, lighter-colored ring; and an outer erythematous ring. (7) In some instances, these lesions may appear with only 2 rings and lack the outermost ring. (8) The dusky appearance to the center of the lesions in urticaria multiforme can appear similar to the target lesions of erythema multiforme; however, the lesions of urticaria multiforme do not have central necrosis or blistering. In addition, erythema multiforme lesions are fixed and may involve oral and other mucous membranes, which is typically not seen in urticaria multiforme. (1)(7)

Serum sickness is a type 3 hypersensitivity (immune complex–mediated) reaction in response to exposure to nonhuman antigens in the serum, which may lead to the development of fever, rash, and arthralgia. (9) Serum sickness–like reactions are often due to medication or vaccine exposure and may present with similar clinical features as serum sickness. The pathophysiology of serum sickness–like reaction has not been well-defined; however, it is not dependent on immune complex deposition, and blood complement levels are typically normal. (10)(11) Both serum sickness–like reactions and urticaria multiforme may have angioedema of the face, hands, and feet, although these features are more common of urticaria multiforme than of serum sickness–like reaction. Clinical features such as high-grade fever, arthralgia, and lymphadenopathy are more often present in serum sickness–like reaction than in urticaria multiforme. (1)(10)(11)

An important clinical feature of urticaria multiforme distinct from either erythema multiforme or serum sickness–like reaction is the transient nature of the lesions in urticaria multiforme. Although the rash of urticaria multiforme may persist for up to 2 weeks, the rash is migratory, and individual lesions will typically resolve within 24 hours. (1)(3) In addition, dermographism is commonly present in urticaria multiforme but in neither of these other conditions. On laboratory evaluation, urticaria multiforme may have mild elevations of the inflammatory markers (erythrocyte sedimentation rate and C-reactive protein) as well as mild leukocytosis, but the degree of elevation would be less than expected for rheumatologic, vascular, or serious infectious conditions. (1) Biopsy of urticaria multiforme would appear indistinct from other types of acute urticaria and is not necessary for diagnosis. (12)

Urticaria multiforme is self-limited and typically resolves within 2 to 12 days. In addition to discontinuation of any offending pharmacologic agents, use of combined systemic antihistamines may aid in symptom resolution. Systemic corticosteroids are usually reserved only for severe cases of urticaria multiforme refractory to use of antihistamine combined use. (1)(3)

Our patient had a characteristic rash of urticaria multiforme in the setting of rhinovirus infection and recent amoxicillin use. Because both viral upper respiratory tract infections and amoxicillin have been associated with the development of urticaria multiforme, it is difficult to definitively identify which factor was the trigger. Urticaria multiforme, erythema multiforme, and serum sickness–like reaction can present with similar-appearing rashes; however, careful examination of the rash and associated symptoms can help distinguish between these conditions.

PATIENT COURSE

In the emergency department, the patient received intravenous fluids and acetaminophen. Given the laboratory and clinical findings, he was diagnosed as having urticaria multiforme secondary to rhinovirus infection or amoxicillin exposure. He was treated with diphenhydramine and cetirizine. Within 24 hours, the rash was less erythematous and demonstrated a migratory pattern, with new lesions appearing as old ones resolved. At 48 hours, blood cultures were negative, and the rash continued to improve so the patient was discharged. Four days later, he was afebrile, and the rash completely resolved without any remaining cutaneous scarring or deformities.

Summary

- Urticaria multiforme is benign, although the dermatologic manifestations may be concerning to parents and health-care providers, which can lead to extensive and unnecessary medical evaluation.

- The history and clinical features can discern urticaria multiforme from mimickers such as erythema multiforme and serum sickness–like reaction. Key findings such as coalescing, migratory lesions lacking central necrosis; absence of arthritis and arthralgias; absence of lymphadenopathy; and adequate response to antihistamines can lead one toward the diagnosis of urticaria multiforme.

- Amoxicillin is a commonly used antibiotic in the pediatric population and a common trigger for urticaria multiforme. Therefore, it is important for providers to recognize the clinical features of urticaria multiforme and distinguish it from more concerning conditions that may also present with rash and fever in a young child.

References for this article can be found at
https://doi.org/10.1542/pir.2022-005745.

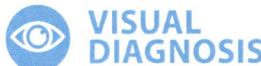

Diffuse Rash in a 10-year-old Boy with Autism

Jessica N. Arvon, BS, * Wesley Lemons, BS,* Chickajajur Vijay, MD,[†] Joseph D. Lynch, MD[†]

*West Virginia University School of Medicine, J.W. Ruby Memorial Hospital, Morgantown, WV

[†]Division of Pediatric Hospital Medicine, Department of Pediatrics, West Virginia University, J.W. Ruby Memorial Hospital, Morgantown, WV

PRESENTATION

A 10-year-old boy with a history of autism who is nonverbal presents to the emergency department with a 2-week history of progressively worsening rash. Per the patient's mother, the rash first appeared on his legs and spread to other parts of his body, including the extensor surfaces of his knees and elbows, as well as to his neck, groin, axillae, and chest (Figs 1–4). The rash is present primarily in photosensitive areas, as he prefers to only wear underwear at home. At first appearance the rash resembled a sunburn, which over time began to dry, crack, and eventually became hyperpigmented. Before presentation to our institution, the patient had been evaluated by his primary care provider, a dermatologist, and had consulted with a different tertiary care center. He had multiple treatment courses during the past 2 weeks, including a week of trimethoprim-sulfamethoxazole and cefalexin, a dose of intramuscular corticosteroid, 3 days of oral fluconazole, and topical treatment with mupirocin and triamcinolone. His mother could not recall the order in which these treatments were tried but did note that they were compliant. She states that none of the medications relieved her son's rash. Despite therapy the rash spread to his forehead and became painful on the areas it covered. He stopped walking secondary to pain from the rash. His mother denies he has any fever, changes in mental status, vomiting, diarrhea, trauma, or new exposures (foods/creams/soaps/detergents). She notes that her son's diet is limited and consists almost exclusively of chicken nuggets. She also states that he is usually naked or in underwear at home. There have been no sick contacts, and no one who has been around him has developed the same rash. Skin examination and punch biopsy reveal the diagnosis.

DIAGNOSIS

The distribution in photosensitive areas and the nature of the rash was suspicious for niacin deficiency. Skin biopsy revealed hyperkeratosis, confluent parakeratosis, pale keratinocytes in the epidermis, and superficial perivascular lymphocytic inflammatory infiltrate. These findings were consistent with nutritional deficiency, especially in the context of an extremely limited diet. Other causes of photodermatoses were considered, the most likely being either drug-induced photosensitivity or phytophotodermatitis (which can occur after exposure to certain plants) given that the patient was taking multiple antibiotics and corticosteroids before admission and could have reasonably been exposed to lemons, limes, celery, or parsley, all of which can cause phytophotodermatitis.

AUTHOR DISCLOSURE: Ms Arvon, Mr Lemons, and Drs Vijay and Lynch have disclosed no financial relationships relevant to this article. This commentary does not contain a discussion of an unapproved/investigative use of a commercial product/device.

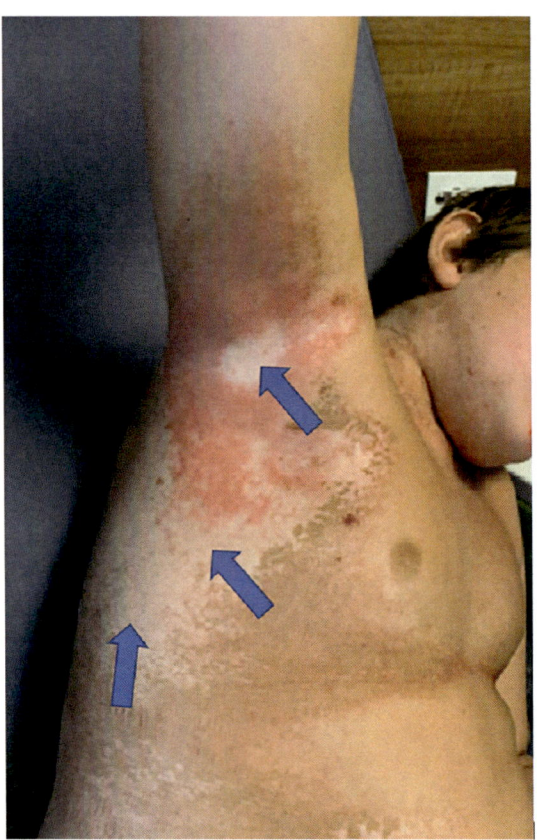

Figure 1. Patient presenting with a hyperpigmented, painful, photosensitive rash. Blue arrows note sparing of the axilla and the area normally covered by an adducted arm.

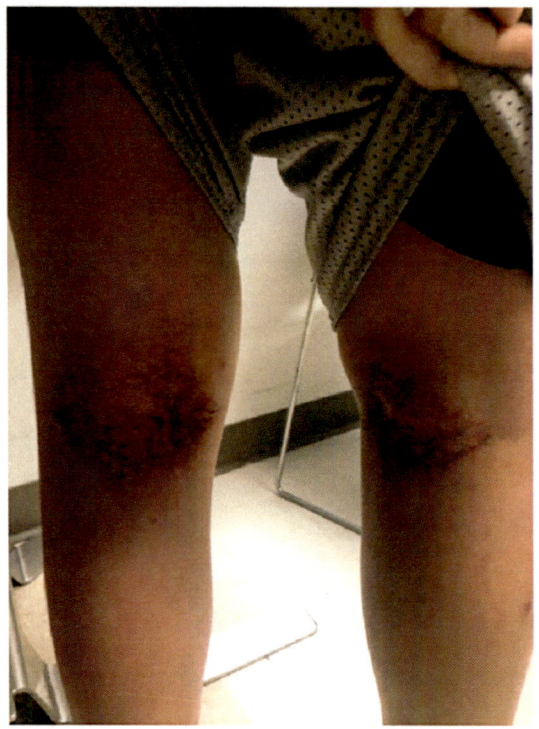

Figure 2. Photosensitive rash bilaterally on the extensor surface of the knees.

Lupus, dermatomyositis, and porphyria were other considerations but were thought to be unlikely given his symptoms.

DISCUSSION

Pellagra is caused by niacin (vitamin B_3) deficiency, which leads to clinical manifestations in the gastrointestinal tract, skin, and nervous system. (1)(2)(3) Pellagra is characterized by the signs and symptoms referred to as the 4 D's: diarrhea, dermatitis, dementia, and eventually death. (4) This devastating sequela results because of niacin's role as a precursor for several coenzymes that regulate cellular metabolism. (1) Due to its key role in cellular metabolism, niacin deficiency tends to affect highly metabolic and regenerative tissues, which explains its predilection to manifest in the skin, brain, and gastrointestinal tract. (5) Niacin is derived from tryptophan, and its synthesis requires vitamins B_2 and B_6. Thus, a deficiency of niacin or its precursor, tryptophan, can result in the classic presentation of pellagra.

Niacin is mainly obtained through meats, legumes, and fish. It is found in large quantities in milk and eggs but is not found in cereals and corn. (6)(7) Malnutrition and tryptophan-deficient corn-based diets are common causes of niacin deficiency. (6)(7)

Studies have shown that the most sensitive manifestation of pellagra is a photosensitive erythematous rash, as was the case in our patient. (8) Dementia and diarrhea show lower specificity. (8) The characteristic skin rash has a photosensitive distribution with well-defined borders, mostly observed on the face, neck (so-called Casal necklace, Fig 4), dorsal surface of the hands, and extensor surface of the forearms. (1)(2)(3) Gastrointestinal symptoms may include diarrhea, stomatitis, and glottis. (9) Neurologic involvement, termed *pellagrous encephalopathy*, may present as memory loss, disorientation, depression, or delirium. Stupor and death may result if untreated. (3)(10)

Diagnosing niacin deficiency or pellagra starts with identifying the characteristic rash and obtaining a dietary history. Skin biopsy and vitamin levels can help exclude other diagnoses being considered but themselves are not diagnostic. Response to niacin supplementation confirms the diagnosis. On microscopic examination, there is "pallor and extensive ballooning of keratinocytes particularly in the upper third of the epidermis with hyperkeratosis in the epidermis." (11) These microscopic changes grossly present as

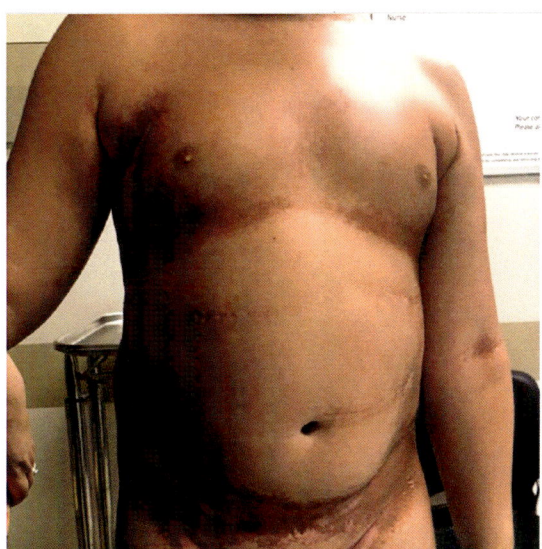

Figure 3. Photosensitive, painful rash covering the anterior abdomen and groin.

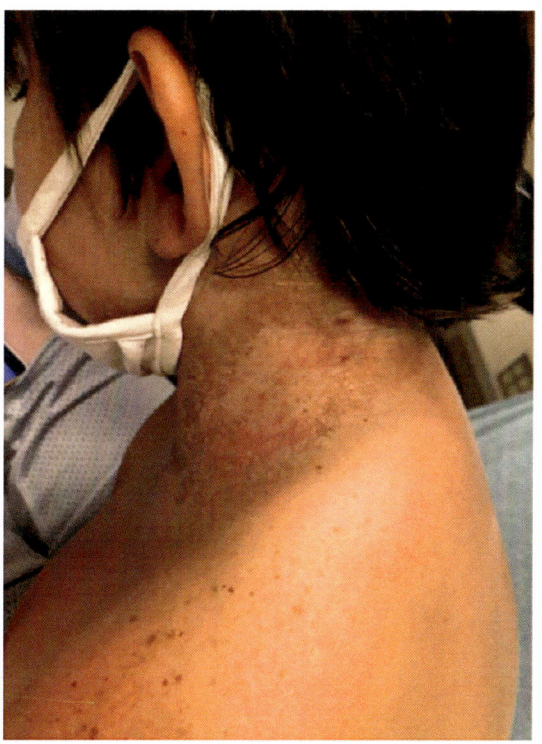

Figure 4. Photosensitive rash around the neck. Note the similar distribution as in Casal necklace.

blister formation and resemble severe sunburn. (11) The keys to diagnosing our patient included his rash, limited diet, skin biopsy, and response to niacin supplementation. Our patient's predilection for not wearing clothes led to a wider distribution of the rash than is usually seen.

Autism spectrum disorder can increase the risk of nutritional deficiency, including pellagra, secondary to selective food intake. Diets limited by textural choices, food color, or other sensory issues can limit the intake of vital nutrients. Our patient had a selective diet of solely chicken nuggets due to his sensitivity to textures of many other foods.

Niacin deficiency is not commonly seen in developed nations after public health implementation of fortified food products. (12) Without a high index of suspicion, the rash can be missed, leading to the previously mentioned sequelae of diarrhea, dermatitis, dementia, and eventual death. Therefore, it is essential that this diagnosis is considered in a subgroup of patients, specifically those with neuropsychiatric disorders leading to food selectivity.

PATIENT COURSE

Multiple sources of nutritional deficiency were investigated, including niacin, folic acid, zinc, and vitamins A, B_6, B_{12}, C, and D. Zinc, folic acid, and niacin levels were found to be low. Our patient had normal calcium levels throughout admission, and radiographs of the femurs excluded rickets, which was considered given his low vitamin D intake. Nutritional rehabilitation and niacin, zinc, and folic acid supplementation were started, in addition to a daily multivitamin while our patient was admitted to the hospital. Nutritional rehabilitation included a balanced diet with a variety of foods (1 fruit, 1 vegetable, and 1 grain on each tray in addition to the patient's chosen protein) offered and encouraged to be consumed, supplemental nutrition with PediaSure® (Abbott Nutritional Products, Abbott Park, IL) with meals, and occupational therapy to work with the patient regarding his oral aversion. He tolerated the supplements without issue but struggled with trying new foods, and the rash became less painful and began to involute. He continued to improve during the next few days. The medical team discussed with his mother the importance of continuing to offer new foods with every meal in addition to continuing his vitamin supplementation at home. Regular appointments were set up with his primary care provider and occupational therapy before discharge. Five weeks after discharge, his skin was clear and pain free following supplementation despite the patient maintaining his same selective diet. Our patient's primary care provider continued to address his selective eating through regular occupational therapy and continued meal variety with encouragement to try new foods.

Summary

- Vitamin deficiencies are relatively rare in developed countries. However, patients with oral aversion, sensory issues, food pickiness, and/or intellectual disabilities are at risk for deficiencies if their diets are not diverse.

- Skin manifestations of pellagra are key to diagnosis and include a photosensitive rash with well-defined borders on the face, neck, and extensor surfaces. (10)(11)(13)

- A high index of suspicion is required to make this diagnosis and help prevent unnecessary and severe neurologic sequelae, including death if left untreated.

References for this article can be found at https://doi.org/10.1542/pir.2021-005226.

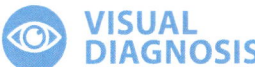

Out of the Blue (Belly)

Ryan Mitacek, MD,* Youmna Mousattat, MD*†

*Charleston Area Medical Center Women and Children's Hospital, Charleston, WV
†West Virginia University School of Medicine, Charleston, WV

PRESENTATION

A 9-year-old girl without chronic medical conditions is brought to the emergency department for a complaint of diffuse abdominal pain and new-onset diffuse abdominal blue discoloration of the skin. She was diagnosed 11 days previously as having a urinary tract infection after 2.5 weeks of dysuria and completed a 7-day course of trimethoprim-sulfamethoxazole with resolution of symptoms. She has no history of allergies or reaction with previous courses of trimethoprim-sulfamethoxazole. On waking the morning of presentation she noticed that her abdomen was bluish in color with diffuse abdominal pain, spreading and intensifying in color throughout the day. The discoloration spread to her back and thighs, with associated spread of pain. The discoloration spares the skin folds and underwear lines. She denies any history of trauma, fevers, nausea/vomiting, upper respiratory tract symptoms, or other rashes. There is no known history of glucose-6-phosphate dehydrogenase or reactions to previous antibiotics. No personal, family, or close contact history of similar skin discolorations is disclosed.

Vital signs on presentation are as follows: temperature, 97.9°F (36.6°C); heart rate, 95 beats/min; blood pressure, 98/74 mm Hg; respiratory rate, 18 breaths/min; and persistently stable oxygen saturations greater than 96%. Evaluations in the emergency department are inconclusive; the only abnormality is a mild elevation in the erythrocyte sedimentation rate at 25 mm/hr. All other evaluations are normal, including complete blood cell count, coagulation studies, urinalysis, cultures, complete metabolic profile, and inflammatory markers. In addition, contrast-enhanced computed tomography of the abdomen is ordered for concern of possible appendicitis or abdominal catastrophe and shows no abnormalities. Co-oximetry and blood gas analysis are not performed. The emergency department orders a 20-mL/kg bolus of normal saline, cefepime, and vancomycin. The general pediatric service is consulted for admission. Physical examination shows a symmetrical patch of blue-purple discoloration over the abdomen, bilateral flanks, and bilateral thighs that spares the skin folds and without any secondary lesions (Fig. 1). There is significant pain on minimal palpation of discolored skin, and the patient refuses to allow attempts at wiping the affected skin with a wet cloth. No axillary or pubic hair is appreciated, and she has Tanner stage 1 breasts. She is admitted to the hospital for intractable pain. While the patient is asleep on the first day of admission, the discoloration is wiped away with an alcohol swab but returns after a few hours (Fig. 2). After this, a Wood lamp is used without findings of fluorescent hyphae. Skin culture

AUTHOR DISCLOSURE: Drs Mitacek and Mousattat have disclosed no financial relationships relevant to this article. This commentary does not contain a discussion of an unapproved/investigative use of a commercial product/device.

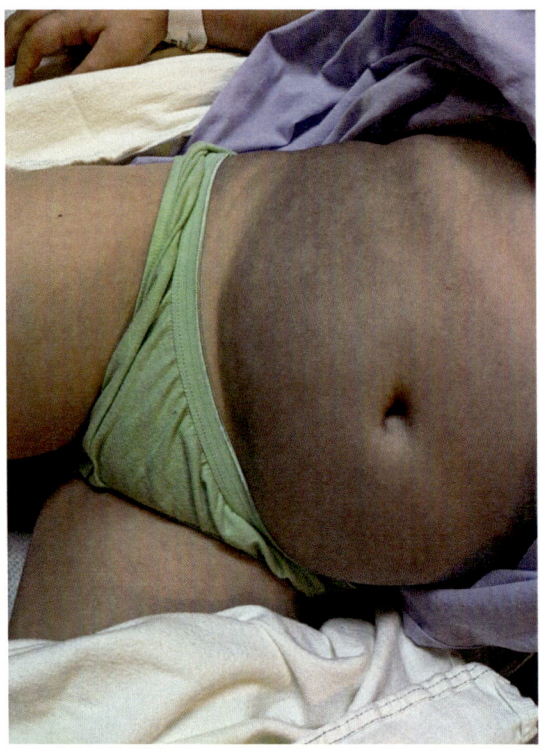

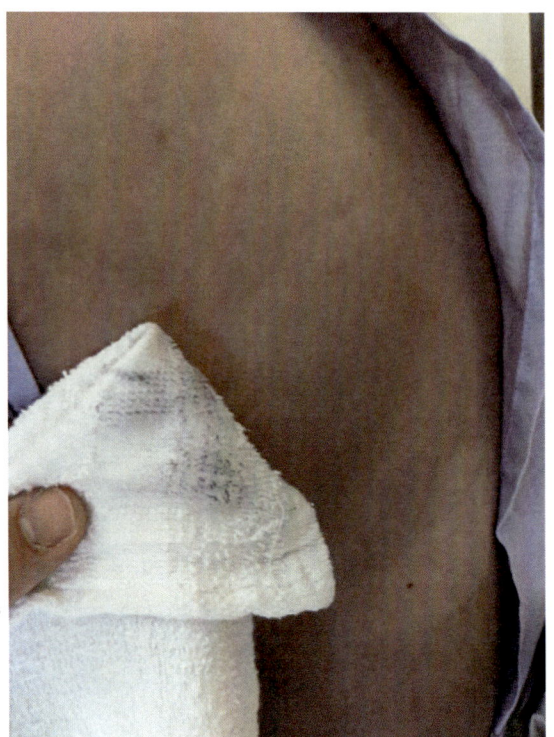

Figure 1. Blue abdominal discoloration that spares the skin folds.

Figure 2. Blue discoloration wiped off with alcohol.

of the pigmented lower abdomen is obtained for concern of infection. Pain is controlled with standard doses of acetaminophen and ibuprofen, and she is discharged with plans for outpatient follow-up. Culture of the skin reveals the diagnosis.

DIAGNOSIS

This child was diagnosed as having pseudochromhidrosis secondary to mold infection. Fungal culture of the skin grew *Penicillium* species.

DISCUSSION

New-onset skin discoloration is a scary condition for both caregivers and providers. The causes of changed color include discolorations of the skin itself, for example cyanosis, hemochromatosis, or the "bronze diabetes" of Addison disease. These can be symptoms of severe systemic illness and require immediate evaluation and treatment. If the discoloration is from outside the skin, the differential diagnosis can include staining of the skin from clothing dyes or discolorations related to sweat. Possible causes of our patient's acquired, diffuse, blue skin discoloration include exogenous ochronosis, drug eruptions, postinflammatory hyperpigmentation, cyanosis, drug reactions (eg, amiodarone and

silver), blue-dyed foods, abdominal trauma, pancreatitis (Grey-Turner sign), retroperitoneal hemorrhage, and medical child abuse (formerly known as Munchausen syndrome by proxy). Pseudochromhidrosis from infectious causes is a condition of uncertain incidence and prevalence. (1) A narrative review from 2020 details only 11 published cases in both the adult and pediatric literature. (2)

Pseudochromhidrosis literally means "false-colored sweat" and refers to the condition of colorless sweat that acquires color after contact with other substances on the skin. It presents as a new-onset discoloration of the skin that can be wiped off with alcohol pads. Colors vary, and blue, red, brown, yellow, and black have been reported. It is a discoloration caused by pigments on the surface of the skin reacting with components of sweat, as opposed to chromhidrosis, which is a discoloration of the sweat itself. There are reports of pain and pruritus with presumed infectious causes. (3) The precise mechanism is unknown but is potentially related to the offending compound directly irritating the skin. Chromhidrosis tends to occur after puberty and in the distribution of the apocrine sweat glands (ie, axillae and groin). Our patient had discoloration predominantly on the abdomen and lower back and was prepubertal without signs of precocious puberty, reducing the pretest probability of chromhidrosis. Other cases of pseudochromhidrosis in similarly aged patients have been reported from bacterial skin infections. (4) Bacterial causes include *Bacillus* species, *Corynebacterium* species, *Serratia marcescens,* and *Pseudomonas aeruginosa*. (2) Other causes include medications, (5)(6) dyes, sunless tanning products, (7) heavy metals, and chemical agents. Fungal infections have been identified as a cause, and a Wood lamp examination can be a useful point-of-care test. (1) Pseudochromhidrosis is a rare entity, and we found no published cases that definitively identified a fungal cause. There is 1 published case that had skin cultures positive for fungi and bacteria. (5) Penicillium species can produce blue pigment when grown on media containing hydrolyzed proteins and salt water, possibly related to the discoloration in our patient. (8) Even pubic lice has been identified as a cause. (9) Detailed evaluation of the skin with a Wood lamp and dermoscope have been found to be useful, possibly showing fluorescence with fungal infection. (10) Our Wood lamp examination was negative, but this may have been a false-negative from the recent cleaning. In addition, this case highlights that a complete skin examination should include attempts at removing discoloration.

Diagnosis is made based on clinical and histologic features and the absence of other causes of skin discoloration. An algorithm for investigation of chromhidrosis and pseudochromhidrosis has been proposed by Tempark et al, (1) with the first 2 steps being to ask for a history of environmental (dyes/chemicals) and medication (eg, topiramate, lansoprazole) exposures. The next step is discontinuation of possible offending medications with skin scraping and culture. If positive for chromogenic bacteria, a diagnosis of pseudochromhidrosis can be made. If negative, a skin biopsy is recommended. If the biopsy is positive for lipofuscin, a diagnosis of chromhidrosis is likely; if negative, pseudochromhidrosis is more likely. (1) Following this algorithm, our patient's positive *Penicillium* species would represent a possible culprit, making a diagnosis of pseudochromhidrosis.

Treatment varies by cause and includes removal of the offending agent. The 2 most recent reviews detail treatments with erythromycin, clindamycin, octenidine, aluminum chloride solution, sulfadiazine, nadifloxacin, sulfamethoxazole-trimethoprim, and/or cefcapene. Most patients received combination topical and oral erythromycin for 1 to 2 weeks with resolution of symptoms. (1)(2) Given the lack of published literature for the treatment of fungal pseudochromhidrosis, we propose using an oral antifungal targeting the identified fungus (eg, fluconazole or itraconazole).

PATIENT COURSE

No bacteria grew from the skin culture, but 3 weeks after hospital discharge the fungal culture of the skin grew *Penicillium* species. The genus *Penicillium* comprises approximately 225 species found in soil, wood, and decaying vegetation. *Penicillium chrysogenum* can cause skin reactivity and colonize the airways of patients with respiratory allergies. Human flora biodiversity studies have identified *P chrysogenum* and *Penicillium lanosum* as normal human flora. (11) Some *Penicillium* species are known to be opportunistic pathogens in the immunocompromised, despite low pathogenicity. (12) Although our patient's preceding treatment with trimethoprim-sulfamethoxazole may have caused alterations in mucocutaneous flora, the authors were unable to find studies identifying a link between trimethoprim-sulfamethoxazole and *Penicillium* species colonization.

Fluconazole was prescribed with guidance from an infectious disease specialist. She did not attend her planned follow-up visit with primary care, and multiple attempts to contact her parents by phone were unsuccessful. A certified letter with a prescription for fluconazole was mailed to the parents.

Summary

- A thorough evaluation of skin discoloration should include an attempt to wipe the color with an alcohol pad.

- Underlying causes of discolored sweat are myriad, and cultures from the skin should be sent for laboratory testing if there is concern for a possible infectious etiology.

- Pseudochromhidrosis and chromhidrosis must be included on the list of differential diagnoses of patients with new-onset skin discoloration.

References for article can be found at
https://doi.org/10.1542/pir.2021-005295.

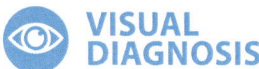

A Frequently Missed Diagnosis of a Firm, Blue-Tinged Mass

Kyung Woo Hong,* David Saulino, DO,† Jessica Ching, MD,‡ Puneet Tung, DO*

*Department of Pediatrics,
†Department of Pathology, and
‡Department of Plastic Surgery, University of Florida, Gainesville, FL

PRESENTATION

An otherwise healthy 5-year-old girl presents to the outpatient pediatric clinic for evaluation of a left temporal mass that has been slowly growing for the past month. The mass is nonpruritic, mildly tender to the touch, and not associated with drainage. There is no recent history of local trauma, including insect bites or scrapes. There is no family history of similar lesions or other skin disorders. Physical examination reveals a solitary 0.4 × 0.6-cm papule that is firm, mildly tender to the touch, and skin-colored to a faint blue–maroon color on the left side of her temple (Fig 1). The remainder of her physical examination findings are normal. She is referred to pediatric dermatology for evaluation and consultation. A clinical diagnosis is made, with dermatology consultation further supporting the diagnosis through dermatoscopy. Treatment options were presented, and the family elected to observe the lesion for several months before proceeding with a surgical referral.

Five months later she presents for her 6-year-old annual wellness physical examination. At this point the left temporal papule has enlarged to a 1.0 × 1.5-cm dark-blue nodule (Fig 2). She is referred to pediatric plastic surgery for consultation of its removal and histopathologic confirmation. In the following month, the nodule is successfully removed and sent for surgical pathologic examination, which confirms the diagnosis.

DIAGNOSIS

The presence of a slowly enlarging, firm, blue-telangiectatic lesion and central white and gray-blue lesion on dermatoscopy (Fig 3) suggests the diagnosis of pilomatrixoma, with confirmation through histopathologic analysis (Fig 4).

DISCUSSION

Pilomatrixoma, also known as pilomatricoma or calcifying epithelioma of Malherbe, is a benign skin tumor of the hair follicle matrix and is of ectodermal origin. It was initially termed "epithelioma" because Malherbe believed that the cell of origin was sebaceous. (1) They are most common in hair-bearing regions, including the head and neck. (2)(3) It occurs in a bimodal pattern with prevalence in childhood but also has been seen in the fifth decade of life. It is most commonly found in the pediatric population, with the mean age at onset being 4.5 years and a mildly higher prevalence in females and in white populations. (3) The exact etiology of its development is unknown but has been associated with trauma,

AUTHOR DISCLOSURE: Mr Hong and Drs Saulino, Ching, and Tung have disclosed no financial relationships relevant to this article. This commentary does not contain a discussion of an unapproved/investigative use of a commercial product/device.

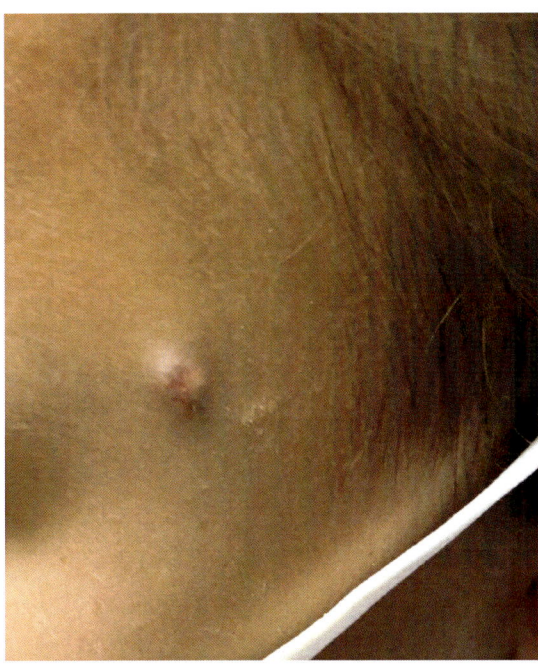

Figure 1. A 0.4 × 0.6-cm skin-colored to faint blue–maroon papule on the left side of the temple at initial presentation.

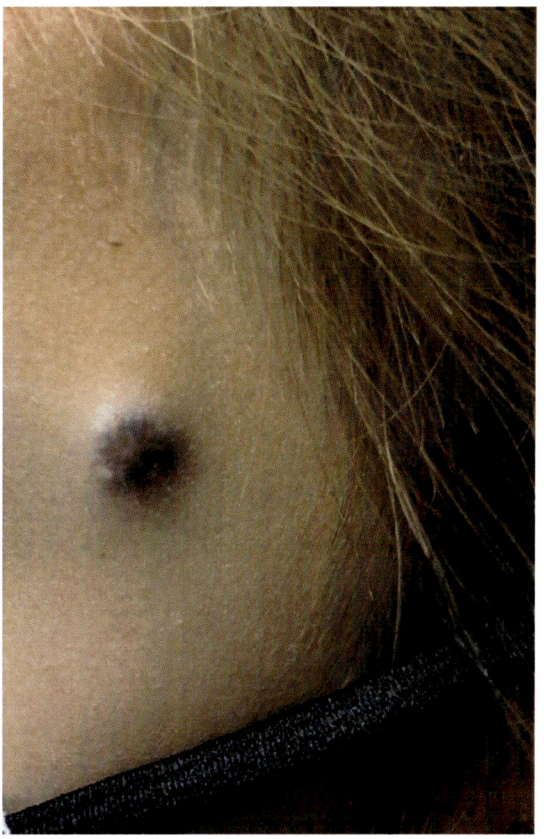

Figure 2. An enlarged 1.0 × 1.5-cm dark-blue nodule seen at a wellness visit 5 months after initial presentation.

surgery, and a mutation in the β-catenin gene, which plays an important role in differentiation of the hair follicle. (1)(4)

The lesion is usually solitary, irregular, firm, mobile, and slowly enlarging over time with a blue or telangiectatic coloration. (5) The mean size of the lesion is 1.2 cm, with a range of 1.0 to 1.5 cm, although there have been reported cases that are larger. (3) Pilomatrixomas are typically asymptomatic, but they may be tender. Ulceration occurs infrequently. (6) A previously described pathognomonic sign for pilomatrixoma is the "tent sign," which is revealed by stretching the skin over the lesion to feel the irregular surface of the lesion. (6)(7) There is no associated lymphadenopathy. Dermatoscopy findings of irregular white structures or ultrasonography findings of well-defined oval mass with internal echogenic foci may be used to further support the clinical evaluation. (4)

Complications of pilomatrixomas are rare, with a malignant version of pilomatrixoma called "pilomatrix carcinoma" having been reported only in the adult population. (8) However, pilomatrixoma has been associated with several syndromes, including myotonic dystrophy, familial adenomatous polyposis–related syndromes (ie, Gardner), and Turner, Sotos, Kabuki, and Rubinstein-Taybi syndromes. (3)(7)(9) Suspicion of underlying syndromes should be raised in patients who present with 6 or more pilomatrixomas, a family history of the associated syndromes or of pilomatrixomas, and a

clinical history suggestive of Turner or Rubinstein-Taybi syndrome (ie, intellectual disability, short stature, premature ovarian failure). (9) In a comprehensive review by Ciriacks et al, (9) only 4.5% of individuals with no underlying syndromes developed more than 5 pilomatrixomas, with 46.3% of individuals with underlying syndromes developing 6 or more. Using the number of pilomatrixomas (≥6) as a screening tool for underlying association

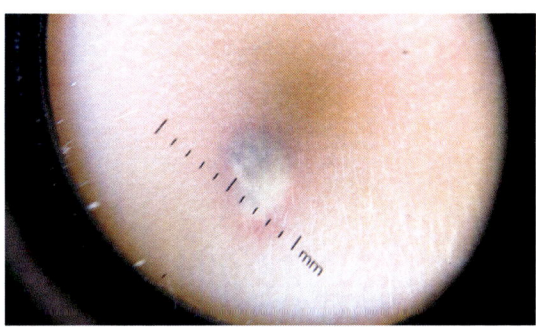

Figure 3. Dermatoscopy showing a 0.4 × 0.6-cm central white to gray-blue lesion with surrounding erythema.

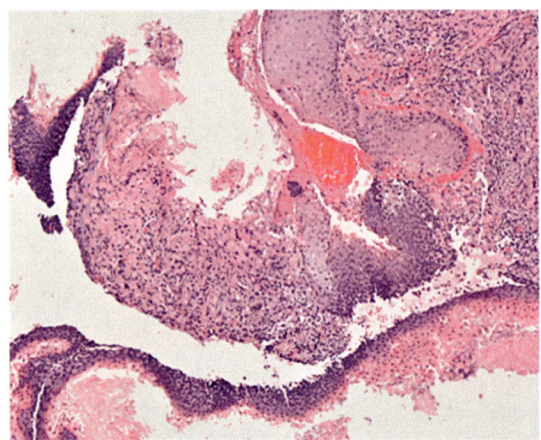

Figure 4. Hematoxylin-eosin slide showing a transition from basaloid cells to anucleate ghost cells with some associated histiocytic inflammation (original magnification ×100).

calcifications). The lesion may be confirmed by histologic analysis if not clinically apparent. (7) Histologic features include basaloid cells transitioning to anucleate epithelial ghost cells along with abundant histiocytic inflammation. These cells can often progress to calcification, leading to the typical firm consistency of the lesion. (5) Fine needle aspirates have been previously used but may lead to false-negatives because ghost cells might not be captured; it can have a diagnostic probability as low as 28%. (10)

No treatment is necessary if the pilomatrixoma is asymptomatic. However, complete surgical excision is the treatment of choice when treatment is indicated (patient's preference, tender, increasing in size, or in a visible location). This may be done with local anesthesia or in the operating room under general anesthesia, depending on the size, location, and patient factors. An incision is made around the lesion and the involved skin, and careful dissection continues circumscribing the mass until is it completely free from the surrounding tissue. The wound bed is inspected to ensure that no residual pilomatrixoma remains. The area is generally closed primarily after undermining local tissue for mobility. Postsurgical recurrence is low (2%–6%) and is mostly associated with inadequate surgical resection. (1)(3)

allows for high specificity (95.5%) and high positive predictive value (80.7%) with the limitation of low sensitivity (46.3%). (9)

Pilomatrixoma is often misdiagnosed, and clinical accuracy ranges from 12.5% to 55.5%. (1)(2)(5)(7) The most likely reason this lesion is misdiagnosed is due to underrecognition. Other potential reasons include the broad differential diagnosis that accompanies benign dermatologic lesions (Table) and the variation in clinical presentation (ie, multiple lesions, atypical locations, or absence of characteristic clinical appearance or

PATIENT COURSE

The patient has been seen 10 days postoperatively by pediatric plastic surgery with no complications and excellent cosmesis.

Table. Differential Diagnosis of Pilomatrixoma

DIFFERENTIAL DIAGNOSIS	CLINICAL EXAMINATION	MANAGEMENT
Epidermal cyst: keratin-filled cyst	Usually mobile, firm, painless, flesh-colored nodule that is common on the face, neck, chest, and genitals.	If asymptomatic, does not require treatment. If symptomatic, infected, or inflamed, can perform total surgical excision.
Dermoid cyst: true hamartoma consisting of skin, hair follicles, and sweat glands	Pathognomonic finding includes protruding hair from dermoidlike cyst. Typically, firm, painless, flesh-colored nodule that is common on the head and neck.	Typically treated with total surgical excision to prevent infection, and adhesion or erosion to underlying bone.
Osteoma cutis: bone formation in the dermis	Painless, single or multiple, firm nodule with 4 variants: isolated, widespread, multiple miliary, and platelike. Presents commonly on the face and scalp.	Perform laboratory evaluation to rule out metabolic abnormality. Can use topical tretinoin in small nodules with surgical excision or lasers (erbium:YAG or carbon dioxide) as mainstay treatments.
Blue nevus: thought to be from failure of migration to the epidermis of neural crest melanocytes	Presents as a smooth-surface, well-demarcated nodule that does not grow in size and is commonly on the face and extremities.	Can monitor stable lesions. If nodules increase in size, can biopsy. For curative care, perform surgical excision.
Venous malformation: venous dilation from smooth muscle cell dysfunction	Light to dark blue subcutaneous skin lesion that is soft and compressible. Persistent thrombi can present as a firm lesion due to calcification/phleboliths. Common on extremities, trunk, neck, and face.	Supportive therapies include compression and pain control. Sclerotherapy, surgery, or sirolimus have been used for curative therapies.

Adapted from multiple references: (1)(3)(11)(12)(13).

In a follow-up phone call 1 month later, the parent stated that she was doing very well and had no concerns.

ACKNOWLEDGMENTS

We thank the interdisciplinary providers listed in the care of our patient; Jessica Allen Ching, MD, for review of the manuscript and the curative procedure; and David M. Saulino, DO, for review of the manuscript, the hematoxylin-eosin slide, and histopathologic confirmation.

Summary

- The differential diagnosis for a solitary, benign skin lesion is broad and leads to a high misdiagnosis of pilomatrixoma (Table). (3)

- Clinical familiarity and suspicion of pilomatrixoma is needed to pursue additional investigation for confirmatory diagnosis and overall prognosis.

- Patients who present with 6 or more pilomatrixomas should be evaluated for an underlying syndrome. (9)

- Histologic features include basaloid cells transitioning to anucleate ghost cells along with abundant histiocytic or granulomatous inflammation.

- Surgical treatment is curative, with a low recurrence rate.

- Complications of pilomatrixoma are rare but include pilomatrix carcinoma, which occurs in the adult population with the tendency to reoccur. (8)

References for this article can be found at
https://doi.org/10.1542/pir.2021-005149.

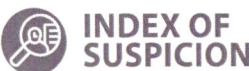

INDEX OF SUSPICION

Hives and Fever in a 13-year-old Boy

Thang V. Truong, MD,*[†] Blake Gruenberg, MD,[‡] Daisy A. Ciener, MD, MS,[‡] Ryan Butchee, MD*

*The Children's Hospital at OU Medical Center, Oklahoma City, OK
[†]University of Iowa Hospitals and Clinics, Iowa City, IA
[‡]Vanderbilt University Medical Center, Nashville, TN

PRESENTATION

A 13-year-old previously healthy immunized boy presents to the pediatric emergency department (ED) with fever, hives, and red-colored urine. He had no history of anaphylaxis, but earlier that morning he had an episode of angioedema, hives, and difficulty breathing. His mother treated him with 25 mg of oral diphenhydramine and 0.3 mg of intramuscular epinephrine obtained from a sibling with a history of anaphylaxis. All of his symptoms improved by the time emergency medical services arrived so he was not transported to a hospital. A couple of hours later he presented to his pediatrician due to recurrence of hives. He was prescribed hydroxyzine and a prednisolone course for presumptive allergic reaction symptoms. That night (12 hours after intramuscular epinephrine administration), his hives were still visible but much improved according to his mother. However, he became febrile to 101.9°F (38.8°C) and also noticed red-colored urine, so he presented to the ED. He did not have nausea, vomiting, or diarrhea. On arrival his vital signs are remarkable for hypoxia to 88% requiring oxygen at 2 L/min via nasal cannula and hypertension to 150/100 mm Hg. On physical examination he appears uncomfortable from pain and has mild diffuse urticaria. He also has 2 dusky lesions on his abdomen surrounded by areas of erythema that are distinctly different from his urticarial rash (Fig 1). These lesions are tender to palpation, but the rest of his abdomen is soft, nontender, and nondistended. He does not have any respiratory distress, wheezing, or angioedema. Initial laboratory values (refer to Table 1 for normal values) are notable for a low platelet count of 100,000/μL (100 × 10⁹/L) and a low hemoglobin level of 11 g/dL (110 g/L). The reticulocyte count is elevated at 10.6% of red blood cells (RBCs) (0.11 proportion of RBCs), and the lactate dehydrogenase level is elevated at 3,934 U/L (65.7 μkat/L). The peripheral blood smear shows that 25% of RBCs are schistocytes. Also notable are elevated levels of blood urea nitrogen of 34 mg/dL (12.1 mmol/L) and creatinine of 1.5 mg/dL (132.6 μmol/L). The coagulation profile is abnormal, with a high international normalized ratio of 1.9, a high D-dimer value of 5,781 μg/mL (31,657 nmol/L), and a prolonged activated partial thromboplastin time of 39 seconds. The white blood cell count is elevated at 24,000/μL (24 × 10⁹/L), and the lactate dehydrogenase level is normal at 302 U/L (5.0 μkat/L). A urine sample appears as shown in Figure 2. After receiving the sample, the laboratory reports that his urine remains pigmented despite multiple centrifugations and that a supernatant cannot be separated. Therefore, dipstick and microscopy results cannot be reported that night using the available colorimetric urine analyzers. The urine myoglobin level,

AUTHOR DISCLOSURE: Drs Truong, Gruenberg, Ciener, and Butchee have disclosed no financial relationships relevant to this article. This commentary does not contain a discussion of an unapproved/investigative use of a commercial product/device.

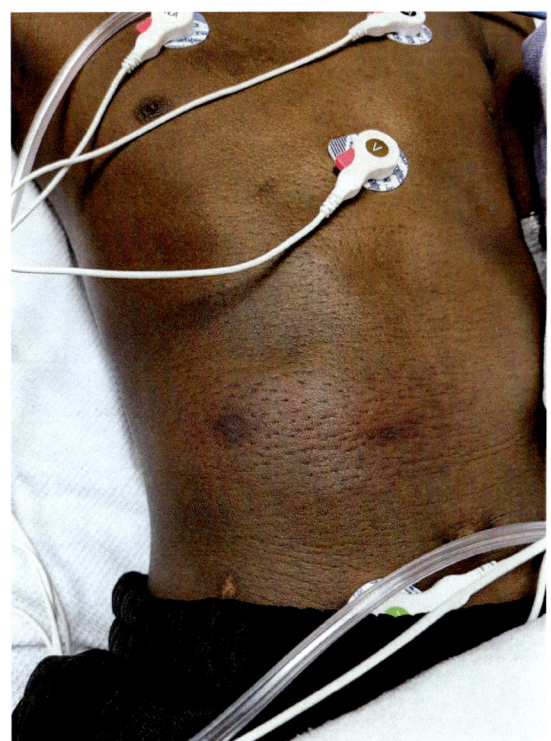

Figure 1. Patient's abdominal skin lesions found on examination at presentation to the emergency department. There are 2 dusky centers surrounded by erythema.

DISCUSSION

Differential Diagnosis

The differential diagnosis for dusky/erythematous skin lesions and red-colored urine includes cellulitis, anaphylaxis, hemolytic uremic syndrome (HUS), Henoch-Schonlein purpura, nephritis syndrome, nephrolithiasis, pyoderma gangrenosum, vasculitis, and systemic loxoscelism (brown recluse spider bite). Although cellulitis can manifest as an erythematous skin lesion, it typically does not have a dusky appearance or result in red-colored urine. The patient does not meet the anaphylaxis criteria while in the ED because he only has hives without respiratory or gastrointestinal involvement. He denies a recent history of bloody diarrhea, making *Escherichia coli* O157: H7–induced HUS unlikely. Nondiarrheal forms of HUS, also known as atypical HUS, are exceedingly rare. Henoch-Schonlein purpura is less likely because the patient does not have purpura or a rash that localized to dependent areas (lower extremities/buttocks). Nephritic syndrome should be considered when hematuria and hypertension are found; however, this does not explain his cutaneous skin findings or evidence of hemolysis on laboratory testing. He denies colicky abdominal or flank pain, making nephrolithiasis less likely. In addition, renal ultrasonography did not show any stones or hydronephrosis. Pyoderma gangrenosum is an idiopathic disorder in which dark erythematous papules progress to necrotic ulcers. The lesion of pyoderma gangrenosum typically is not as well-demarcated and often has ragged, ribbon-like ulcers. (1) It should be suspected in patients with preceding trauma to the area or those who have other systemic illnesses, such as inflammatory bowel disease, juvenile idiopathic arthritis, and other rheumatologic arthritides, or leukemia, none of which is suggested in this patient's history. Similarly, vasculitis is less likely in this patient because he does not have any history of underlying

however, is elevated to 1,962 μg/L (114 nmol/L). Chest radiography is normal. Renal ultrasonography shows increased renal parenchymal echogenicity but no hydronephrosis or stones. At the time of admission, repeated laboratory values are significant for a decreased hemoglobin level of 7.8 g/dL (78 g/L) and an increased creatine kinase level of 645 U/L (11 μkat/L).

Table 1. Normal Laboratory Values in Order of Appearance in Manuscript

LABORATORY TEST	NORMAL VALUES IN CONVENTIONAL UNITS	NORMAL VALUES IN SYSTÈME INTERNATIONAL (SI) UNITS
Platelets	150–400 × 10³/μL	150–400 × 10⁹/L
Hemoglobin	11.4–15.4 g/dL	114–154 g/L
Reticulocyte count	0.5%–2.5% of red blood cells	0.005–0.025 proportion of red blood cells
Lactate dehydrogenase	62–496 U/L	1.0–8.3 μkat/L
Blood urea nitrogen	7–17 mg/dL	2.5–6.1 mmol/L
Creatinine	0.8–1.1 mg/dL	70.7–97.2 μmol/L
International normalized ratio	0.9–1.2	0.9–1.2
D-dimer	<0.24 μg/mL	1.3 nmol/L
Activated partial thromboplastin time	26.0–37.0 s	26.0–37.0 s
White blood cells	4,500–13,500/μL	4.5–13.50 × 10⁹/L
Creatine kinase	58–391 U/L	1.0–6.5 μkat/L
Urine myoglobin	0–13.8 μg/L	0–0.8 nmol/L
Potassium	3.5–5.1 mEq/L	3.5–5.1 mmol/L

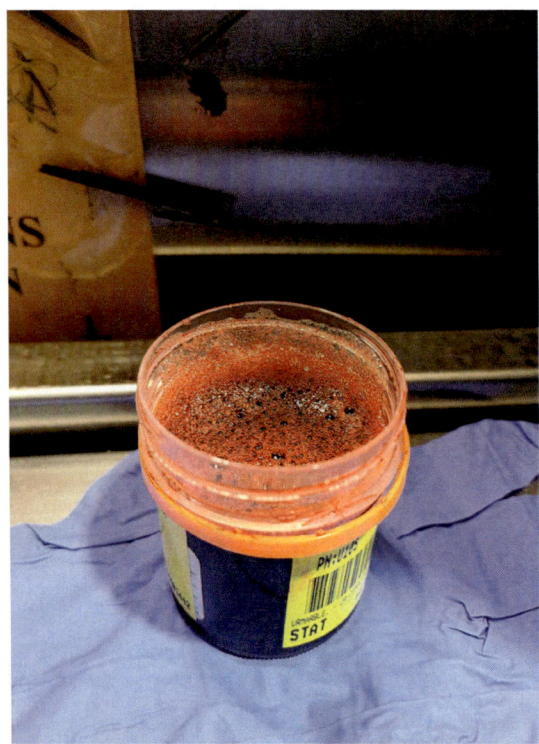

Figure 2. The patient's urine sample obtained in the emergency department.

elastin-degrading metalloproteinases and causes apoptosis of keratinocytes, resulting in neutrophil chemotaxis. (7) Clinically, this manifests as localized pain, necrosis, inflammation, and edema. Interestingly, there is no association between the severity of local tissue damage and the development of systemic symptoms such as fever, emesis, and myalgia. For reasons not yet fully understood, systemic symptoms are relatively more common in children than in adults. (8) In severe cases of systemic loxoscelism, acute hemolysis, disseminated intravascular coagulation (DIC), acute kidney injury (AKI), and rhabdomyolysis can occur. (8)(9) If acute hemolysis is present, it typically occurs within 7 days after local inoculation. (10) Phospholipase D enzyme is also the driving mechanism behind hemolysis via activation of complement pathways. (7)(11) Disseminated intravascular coagulation, characterized by intravascular microthrombi, also causes mechanical shearing of RBCs, further contributing to hemolysis. In addition, the toxin from *L reclusa* causes direct damage to renal tubular epithelial cells, leading to AKI. Free hemoglobin (from hemolysis) and myoglobin (from rhabdomyolysis) also directly damage the renal tubules in a process known as pigmentary nephropathy. (12)(13) The pigmented urine associated with systemic loxoscelism can remain homogenously red/brown due to hemoglobin and myoglobin not separating into a supernatant after centrifugation. In contrast, RBCs can be separated from the rest of the urine specimen into a grossly clear supernatant in which cells are visible under microscopy. (14)(15) AKI, rhabdomyolysis, and acute hemolysis can all lead to life-threatening hyperkalemia.

connective tissue disease, recent infections, or exposure to offending medications.

The Condition and Patient's Diagnosis

This patient has systemic loxoscelism caused by the toxin of *Loxosceles reclusa*, or the brown recluse spider. These spiders are endemic to the midwestern and southern United States. Certain distinguishing features of the brown recluse spider include a violin-shaped print on the anterior thorax as well as 3 pairs of 2 eyes as opposed to the typical 2 pairs of 4 eyes of other arachnid species. (2) As their name implies, they typically live in dark cool spaces inside homes but can also be found outside under dead foliage or logs. (3) Bites are more common from April to October. (4) Brown recluses rarely bite twice, but emerging case reports have reported multiple adjacent inoculations. (5) The initial bite often goes unnoticed as it is typically painless. The bite wound initially manifests as an erythematous macule with subsequent development of a dusky center within 24 hours. The bite wound progresses to central necrosis 10% of the time. (6) Local tissue damage is attributed to the phospholipase D enzyme in the toxin. This enzyme generates potent collagen/

Treatment/Management

Systemic loxoscelism typically resolves in 1 week if no further complications occur. Management of the local bite includes conservative therapy such as cleaning the inoculated area copiously with soap and water, elevating the wound if possible to mitigate localized edema, using cool packs, managing pain, and updating tetanus vaccine if the patient has not received at least 3 doses of tetanus toxoid, with the last dose being administered within the past 10 years. Patients should monitor the wound for progression to necrosis, which typically occurs 10 days after inoculation. (16) No treatment has been proven to halt this progression if it occurs. Corticosteroids, intravenous immunoglobulin, and dapsone have been studied but have not shown consistent efficacy and are not recommended as the standard of care. (17) There is yet to exist an antivenom in the United States. However, one is available in South America as local *Loxosceles* species

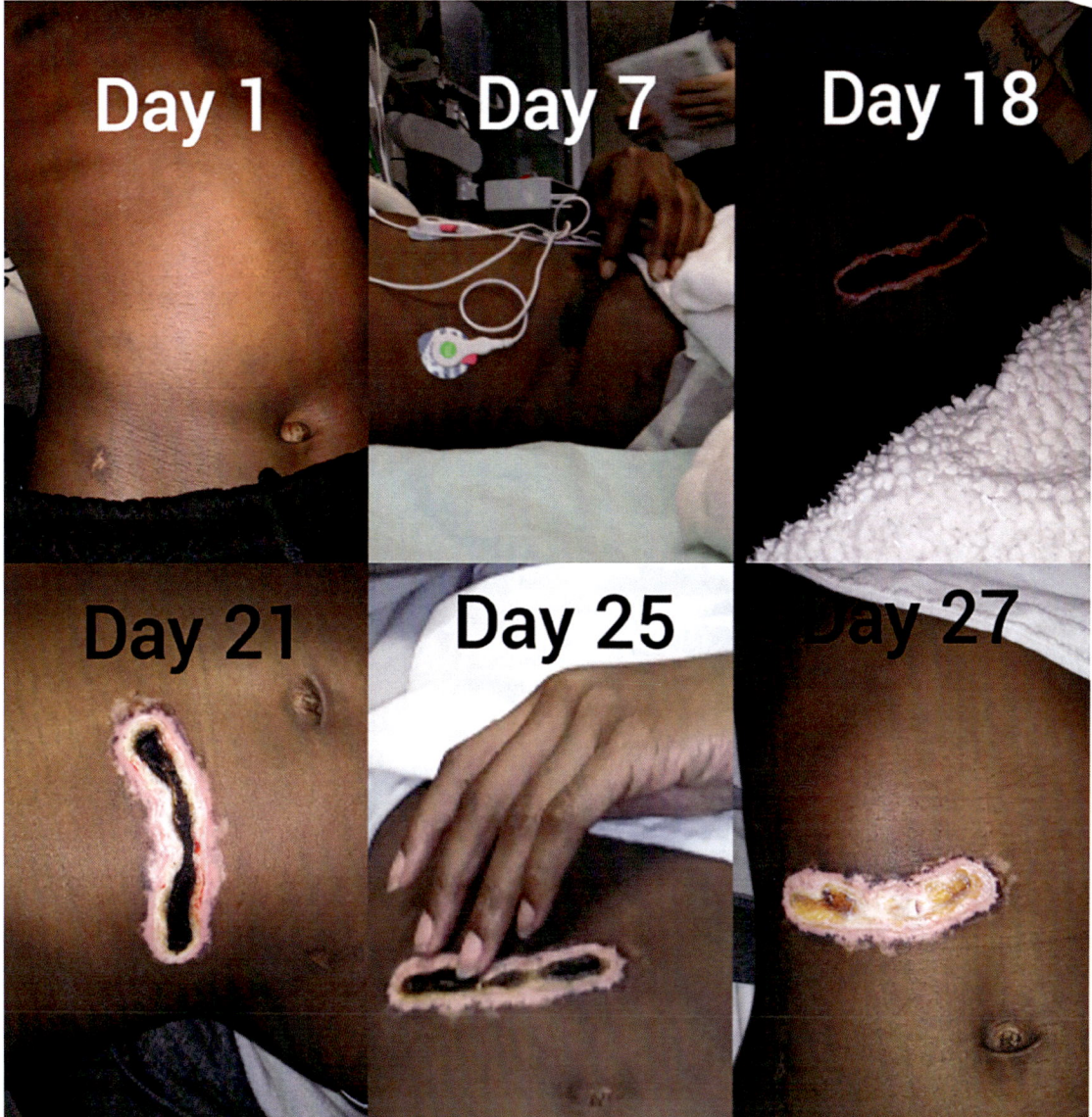

Figure 3. Progression of the patient's skin lesions throughout hospitalization and after discharge. The photograph on day 1 was taken by the patient's mother earlier that day before presentation to the emergency department. Day 7 and day 18 photographs were taken by the medical team during the patient's hospitalization. He was then discharged, and the day 21, 25, and 27 photographs were sent to the medical team by his mother.

(specifically *Loxosceles laeta*) cause a higher incidence of systemic loxoscelism than its North American counterpart *L reclusa*. (18) In North America, therapies are largely supportive for both local and systemic complications of the brown recluse spider bite. Blood transfusion is a cornerstone for patients who are severely anemic or hemodynamically unstable. Plasma exchange has been trialed for severe cases, and consultation with a hematologist is prudent. (19) In children, management of rhabdomyolysis includes the infusion of isotonic saline (targeting a urine output of 4 mL/kg per hour) to mitigate progression to renal failure. (20) AKI, acute hemolysis, and rhabdomyolysis can lead to hyperkalemia and subsequent dysrhythmias, so close monitoring of electrolytes is necessary. Hyperkalemia is initially treated with calcium gluconate/chloride to stabilize the cardiac membrane, followed by albuterol and insulin with glucose to drive potassium intracellularly. Urine alkalization along with diuretics and polystyrene sulfonates can increase renal and gastrointestinal clearance, respectively. Patients with persistent hyperkalemia and AKI with progression to renal failure might require dialysis. Coagulopathy management often includes vitamin K and/or targeted infusion of blood products.

Patient Course

After his initial presentation and resuscitation, the patient was admitted to the PICU. He progressed to severe rhabdomyolysis, hemolysis, hyperkalemia, and dysrhythmia. His potassium level, initially normal in the ED, rapidly increased to 7.1 mEq/L (7.1 mmol/L) in the PICU. In addition, he had the onset of premature ventricular contractions and a widening QRS complex. His hyperkalemia persisted despite treatment with calcium gluconate, albuterol, insulin/glucose, bicarbonate, and diuretics. Due to anticipated progression to life-threatening arrhythmias and cardiac arrest, the PICU team intubated him to facilitate timely and safe dialysis catheter placement. Nephrology was consulted, and he was placed on continuous renal replacement therapy for recalcitrant hyperkalemia and deteriorating renal function. His course was further complicated by hematemesis due to his ongoing thrombocytopenia and coagulopathy. He was given vitamin K and multiple blood product transfusions along with a high-dose proton pump inhibitor. After 2 days he was extubated and transitioned from continuous renal replacement therapy to intermittent dialysis to complete kidney recovery during his 18-day hospital admission. After discharge, his mother continued sharing photos of his abdominal lesions to keep the medical team updated with his healing progress (Fig 3). Wound care therapists continued to follow him as an outpatient until he made a complete recovery.

Lessons for the Clinician

- In severe cases of systemic loxoscelism, acute hemolysis, disseminated intravascular coagulation, acute kidney injury, and rhabdomyolysis can occur.
- There is no association between the severity of local manifestations and the development of systemic symptoms.
- Urine supernatant that remains pigmented after centrifugation is a result of either hemoglobinuria from acute hemolysis or myoglobinuria from rhabdomyolysis. In contrast, hematuria due to hemorrhage in the urinary tract can be separated via centrifugation.
- Corticosteroids, intravenous immunoglobulin, and dapsone have inconsistent efficacy, and their use is not recommended. The standard of care is largely supportive, focusing on the complications of systemic loxoscelism.

References for this article can be found at
https://doi.org/10.1542/pir.2020-003848

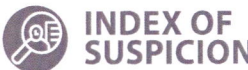

INDEX OF SUSPICION

Rash in a 2-month-old Premature Infant

Margaret Urschler,* Mary Anne Jackson, MD, FAAP, FIDSA, FPIDS,*† Mary Tyson, MD, Barbara Pahud, MD, MPH†

*University of Missouri–Kansas City School of Medicine, Kansas City, MO
†Department of Infectious Diseases, Children's Mercy Hospital, Kansas City, MO

PRESENTATION

An 82-day-old girl presents with a 4-day history of a generalized rash without other systemic symptoms. She was born at 32 weeks' gestation of a dichorionic triamniotic pregnancy. Her neonatal course was uncomplicated, and she was discharged along with her 2 brothers at 47 days of life. The rash began with 1- to 3-mm papules and vesicles on the anterior neck and then spread to her face and scalp over the next 24 hours, with spread of macules, papules, and pustules over the next several days to the chest, torso, and lower extremities (Fig). The infant appears well, is afebrile, is not scratching, and is not irritable. The infant's mother denies exposure to anyone with rash. The infant does not attend child care, but her 4-year-old sibling does. Her parents and siblings report being healthy, and the 2- and 4-year-old siblings are both fully immunized for age per recommended guidelines. Varicella is suspected based on the rash characteristics; her mother reports having had varicella (chickenpox) as a child. The patient is referred to infectious diseases for further evaluation.

Differential Diagnosis

Diagnosis depends on history and physical examination findings to differentiate chickenpox from other diseases associated with vesiculopapular lesions, including rash progression and distribution, the presence of pruritus or pain, exposures, previous varicella or vaccine history, and presence of other systemic features (Table).

Diagnosis

Varicella is traditionally a clinical diagnosis and is easily recognized in the setting of a significant exposure and classic exanthema. In this patient, the diagnosis was more difficult because a specific exposure was not initially ascertained. In most infants beyond 28 weeks' gestation with a positive maternal varicella-zoster virus (VZV) history, one could assume that the newborn is immune via transplacental transfer of antibody; in this case, it seems that the infant had incomplete immunity. Because fewer current clinicians have seen varicella, clinical comfort with diagnosis might be less than in the prevaccine era. Vaccines have decreased the incidence of VZV up to 95%, including an 80% decline in varicella incidence in infants. (1) As a result, not all providers are able to diagnose wild-type VZV because atypical presentations due to vaccination or partial immunity can mimic other diseases. Each year in the United States, VZV vaccination prevents more than 3.5 million cases of chickenpox. (1) Breakthrough

AUTHOR DISCLOSURE: Dr Pahud has been an investigator on clinical trials funded by GlaxoSmithKline and Alios Biopharma/Janssen and has received honoraria from Merck, GlaxoSmithKline, Alios Biopharma/Janssen, Pfizer, Sequiris, and Sanofi Pasteur for service on advisory boards and for nonbranded presentations. Drs Urschler, Jackson, and Tyson have disclosed no financial relationships relevant to this article. This commentary does not contain a discussion of an unproved/investigative use of a commercial product/device.

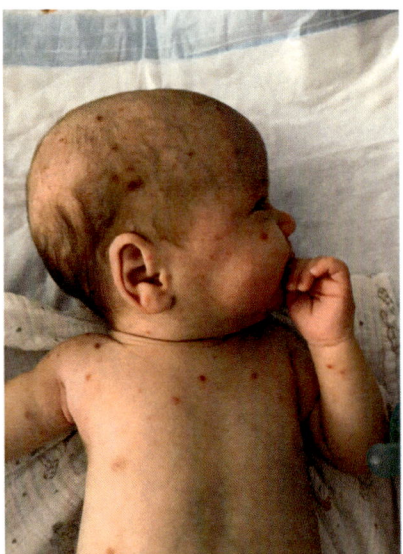

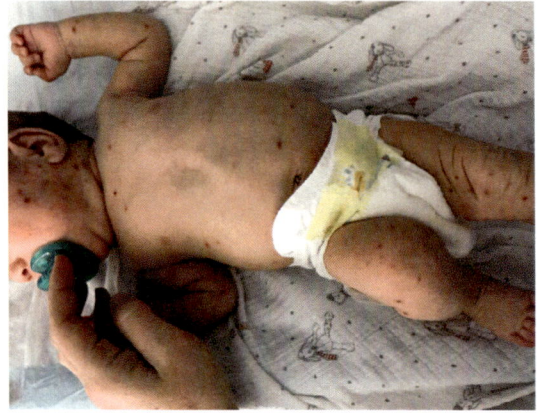

Figure. Photographs of the patient with rash taken on days 2 and 3 after illness onset.

disease after varicella vaccination can occur when VZV disease presents more than 42 days after vaccination; it is often a mild illness with fewer, atypical (maculopapular) skin lesions and a faster recovery. (2)

Polymerase chain reaction of a vesicular lesion or scab is very sensitive and specific for VZV and can distinguish the vaccine strain from the wild-type strain. Immunoglobulin G (IgG) serology assays are available and specific for VZV but have low sensitivity to detect vaccine-induced immunity. (2)

DISCUSSION

Polymerase chain reaction from a skin lesion was obtained for herpes simplex virus and VZV, and testing confirmed VZV infection. The suspected exposure was the patient's mother, who later revealed a history of a dermatomal rash

on her extremity 2 weeks before the infant's presentation. We suspect that the infant's preterm birth and possibly the placental chorionicity (number of placentae in a multiple gestation pregnancy) influenced the presence and magnitude of transplacental varicella antibody, resulting in her mild varicella presentation. IgG transplacental varicella antibody is clearly influenced by gestational age. In this case of a dichorionic triamniotic pregnancy (2 placentas, 3 amniotic sacs), our patient had her own placenta and her brothers shared a placenta. Umbilical cord antibody concentrations are known to be lower in monochorionic twin pregnancies (fetuses share a single placenta) compared with dichorionic twin pregnancies (each fetus has a placenta), theoretically resulting in a higher IgG transfer in our patient, who had her own placenta. (3) However, despite this, our patient was affected by VZV more than her brothers, who shared a placenta. The triplet brothers developed vesicles localized to their scalps about 3 weeks after their sister's infection. Although varicella infection generally confers lifelong immunity, a history of varicella is not a contraindication to vaccination, and vaccination should be considered in all 3 infants because their disease could have been modified by partial immunity that is not fully protective.

The Condition

After exposure, primary varicella occurs in up to 90% of those susceptible after an incubation period of 10 to 21 days. The classic exanthema occurs in 3 to 4 crops of lesions. Macules appear first, followed by papules and vesicles, on the face and scalp and then involving the chest, back, and extremities, with crusting after 4 to 7 days. Complications of primary varicella include bacterial superinfections, pneumonia, encephalitis, thrombocytopenia, or rarely, glomerulonephritis, arthritis, or hepatitis. Herpes zoster (HZ) infection, or shingles, is a reactivation of a latent varicella infection and is characterized by grouped vesicular skin lesions in dermatomal distributions associated with pain and itching. HZ lesions contain active virus, and any susceptible person in contact with the rash blisters is at risk for chickenpox infection. Maternal HZ likely accounts for the patient exposure.

Largely regarded as an invariable and benign infection of childhood, in the prevaccine era nearly all individuals acquired natural infection by adulthood. Complications occurred, and on average 100 children died of varicella each year. If a woman develops primary varicella during the first 20 weeks of pregnancy, congenital varicella, manifest as eye, limb, and neurologic abnormalities, might rarely occur. Since the varicella vaccine was introduced in 1995, there has been a 97% decrease in primary varicella cases. Vaccine coverage is currently greater than 90%, and vaccine immunity occurs in

Table. Differential Diagnosis

DISEASE	RASH	RASH PROGRESSION DISTRIBUTION	EXPOSURE	PRURITUS	PAINFUL LESIONS	OTHER CLUES	DIAGNOSIS
Varicella	Macules, followed by papules, vesicles; crust after 4–7 d	Scalp and face, then chest and torso, then extremities	10–21 d after exposure to varicella or herpes zoster	++	–	In neonate, no maternal history of varicella or varicella vaccine or history of birth before 28–32 weeks' gestation	VZV PCR of skin lesion
HSV	Vesicular cropped lesions	Presenting area and areas of trauma from, eg, scalp electrode	7–14 d after exposure to mother with primary genital herpes at delivery	–	+/–	Can occur after exposure to other contacts with herpes labialis	HSV PCR of skin, blood, and CSF
Scabies	Vesiculopapules	Palms and soles	Adult with typical scabies	++++	–		Skin scraping
Contact dermatitis	Vesicular usually extremities	Area of contact	Psoralen (citrus) or urushiol (poison ivy) plants	+++++	+	Handling limes or outdoor activity	
Atopic dermatitis	Erythema	Face, neck, and extensor surfaces	Vesicles when co-infection with Coxsackie virus or HSV	+++++	++	Family history eczema	Coxsackie virus or HSV PCR from skin lesion
Impetigo	Vesiculopapules	Mouth, face, or diaper area	Others in family with skin abscesses	–	+	*Staphylococcus aureus* or GAS	Bacterial culture skin lesion
Sweet syndrome	Erythematous nodules or plaques (5)	Arms, legs, trunk, face, or neck		–	+++	Consider underlying primary immunologic or genetic disorder	Skin biopsy
Langerhans cell histiocytosis	Vesiculopapules; may resemble seborrhea (6)	Head, neck, ears, diaper area		–	++++	Liver, spleen, bone marrow involvement	Skin biopsy

CSF=cerebrospinal fluid, FH=, GAS=group A *Streptococcus*, HSV=herpes simplex virus, PCR=polymerase chain reaction, VZV=varicella-zoster virus. "+" indicates presence of this symptom, "–" indicates absence of this symptom, and "+/–" indicates symptom may be present or absent.

90% of those immunized with 1 dose of vaccine and in 97% of those with 2 doses; vaccine immunity is long-lasting.

Transplacental transport of IgG antibodies from the pregnant woman to her unborn baby begins at approximately 17 weeks' gestation and continues until close to term. (4) The increase of the fetal IgG concentration between 29 and 41 weeks is double the concentration between 17 and 28 weeks. (4) For VZV specifically, studies have shown that the fetal IgG–maternal IgG concentrations are equal between 32- and 36-weeks' gestation (4) and after birth; these antibodies wane after 3 to 6 months. Premature infants are at increased risk for vaccine-preventable diseases, including VZV, compared with term infants due to decreased transplacental transfer of IgG antibodies. Generally, infants born before 28 weeks are considered susceptible to varicella and those born between 28 and 32 weeks are thought to be at risk because of lower antibody concentrations. (4) Antibodies in term infants may be present for up to 6 months, and, even if present, antibodies wane faster in preterm infants compared with those born at term. (4)

Treatment

Antiviral therapy is not recommended in children with mild disease. Antiviral therapy in the form of acyclovir or valacyclovir is typically reserved for patients at greater risk for moderate to severe disease, including unvaccinated children older than 12 years, those with chronic cutaneous or pulmonary diseases, patients receiving long-term salicylate therapy, or patients receiving courses of corticosteroids or who are otherwise immunocompromised. Supportive therapy for any child with VZV includes keeping fingernails short to prevent trauma from scratching, frequent baths, use of calamine lotion to reduce pruritis, and acetaminophen use if febrile. Aspirin should not be given to these patients due to the risk of Reye syndrome. (2)

Varicella zoster immune globulin should be given for susceptible individuals with significant exposure who pre-sent within a 10-day window if they have an underlying condition that places them at risk for severe complications of varicella. Based on the recommendations in the *Red Book 2021* on the management of exposures to VZV, the 2 triplet siblings would not be candidates for varicella zoster immune globulin. (2) But some experts might recommend preemptive antiviral therapy in this case. In addition, because of the safety of varicella vaccine and the concern that subclinical infection might not confer immunity, immunization of the 2 triplets should be considered.

Lessons for the Clinician

- Varicella-zoster virus and herpes zoster require a high index of suspicion since disease prevalence and incidence have decreased. Laboratory methods are increasingly used to help with diagnosis because clinical recognition of the disease is less common since vaccine introduction.
- When clinicians identify an exposure history, to either primary varicella or shingles, they need to consider whether the patient is susceptible to varicella based on age, vaccination history, and, for premature infants, whether transplacental immunity is likely.
- Premature infants are at risk for varicella because transplacental transport of immunoglobulin G antibodies can be absent in those born before 28 weeks' gestation and inadequate for protection in those born between 28- and 32-weeks' gestation.

Acknowledgments

Thank you to the family for giving permission to present this case and to the Medical Writing Center at Children's Mercy Hospital for their review of this manuscript.

References for this article can be found at
https://doi.org/10.1542/pir.2020-003897

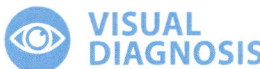
VISUAL DIAGNOSIS

A Child with Swelling and Discoloration of the Fingertip

Sara A. Kullberg, MD,* Ingrid Polcari, MD,† Jeffrey Louie, MD,† Callie Becker, MD†

*Department of Dermatology, School of Medicine, and †Department of Pediatrics, Masonic Children's Hospital, University of Minnesota, Minneapolis, MN

PRESENTATION

A 3-year-old girl with a history of atopic dermatitis presents to the emergency department with sudden onset of swelling and color change of the left third fingertip (Figs 1 and 2). Atopic dermatitis has been previously treated with various modalities, including bleach baths and wet wraps. Her atopic dermatitis is currently active and managed with topical corticosteroids and topical calcineurin inhibitors. The patient's immunizations are up to date. Historical food sensitivities include scrambled eggs (leading to face swelling) and peanut butter (leading to vomiting). On her emergency department physical examination, a tender hemorrhagic bulla is noted on the pad of her left third fingertip. She has no history of underlying trauma, fever, or systemic signs of illness, although notably her mother was recently treated for streptococcal pharyngitis.

Given an unclear etiology of finger swelling, a radiograph is obtained to rule out fracture. The radiograph does not show evidence of bone abnormalities. Two days later she presented again to the emergency department with an additional blister on the pad of her right third fingertip. During her second emergency department visit the bulla on the right hand started draining pus, which was subsequently expressed and cultured.

DIAGNOSIS

Wound culture from the blister on her finger grows methicillin-sensitive *Staphylococcus aureus* and *Streptococcus pyogenes*. Clinical presentation and cultures are consistent with blistering distal dactylitis.

DISCUSSION

Blistering distal dactylitis is primarily a clinical diagnosis, supplemented with a confirmed culture of *Streptococcus* with or without *Staphylococcus* as the underlying organism (group A *Streptococcus* is most common). (1)(2)(3) Group B *Streptococcus* and methicillin-resistant *S aureus* (MRSA) have also been reported as causative agents. (4)(5)(6)(7)(8) A differential diagnosis for similar-appearing entities to consider in this clinical scenario include friction blisters, contact dermatitis, pompholyx, thermal/chemical burns, arthropod bite, bullous impetigo, acute paronychia, and herpetic whitlow. Clinical history, appearance on physical examination, and culture when appropriate should help further distinguish between these entities.

AUTHOR DISCLOSURE Drs Kullberg, Polcari, Louie, and Becker have disclosed no financial relationships relevant to this article. This commentary does not contain a discussion of an unapproved/investigative use of a commercial product/device.

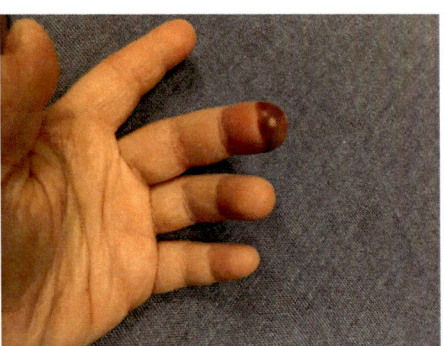

Figure 1. Photograph at the time of initial presentation showing a hemorrhagic, edematous, well-demarcated bulla encompassing the distal pad of the third digit on the left hand.

Blistering distal dactylitis presents as a superficial infection of the volar aspect or finger pad of distal digits, which leads to the development of bullae filled with purulent material. (1)(2)(3) Bullae are hypothesized to develop secondary to significant subepidermal edema, although this mechanism has not been pathologically proved. *S aureus* has a known exfoliative toxin that can cleave desmoglein 1 in the superficial epidermis, although the *Streptococcus* family does not have a similar process that can be attributed to the development of bullae. (1) Regardless of the underlying cause, all forms appear clinically identical to each other.

The most common age range of patients infected is 2 to 16 years, although cases have been seen among newborns and adults, particularly in patients who are immunocompromised. (2)(4)(5)(6)(7)(8)(9)(10)(11)(12) Although Hays and Mullard, (3) who first described blistering distal dactylitis, hypothesized that it classically originates from autoinoculation of the finger due to nose-picking in children, patients can have either associated *Streptococcus* or *S aureus* growth either from elsewhere in the body or from a close contact, and external microbial invasion can occur through open wounds. (2) Atopic dermatitis may be a predisposing risk factor for blistering distal dactylitis because the skin barrier dysfunction inherent to the disease mechanistically increases the risk of cutaneous infection regardless of the type.

If bullae are tense and uncomfortable, they can be treated with either incision and drainage or deflation with a sterile needle and subsequent wet compresses. Systemic antibiotic courses (eg, first-generation cephalosporin) for 7 to 14 days ensuring coverage for both *Streptococcus* and *Staphylococcus* complemented by localized wound care are the standards for treatment. (1)(2)(3) Antibiotic coverage can be tailored based on susceptibility testing. When MRSA is suspected, clindamycin or trimethoprim/sulfamethoxazole should be used empirically depending on local prevalence and susceptibilities of community-acquired MRSA strains. (13) With cases positive for MRSA and associated systemic symptoms, a very rare form of blistering distal dactylitis that has been described in only a few case reports, it is recommended to treat with intravenous vancomycin. (7)(14)

PATIENT COURSE

In the emergency department, drainage from the patient's finger was cultured and she was sent home on 5 days of

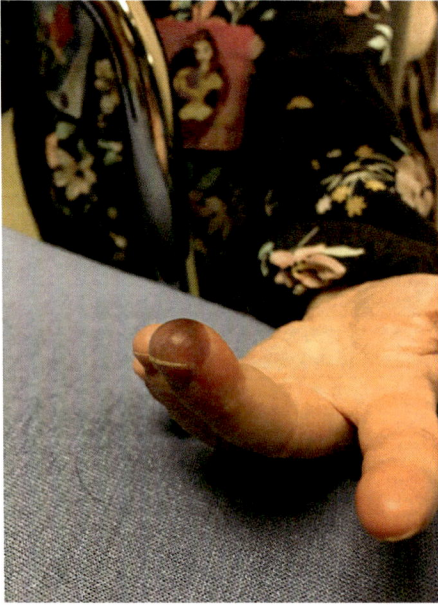

Figure 2. Photograph at the time of initial presentation showing a hemorrhagic, edematous, well-demarcated bulla encompassing the distal pad of the third digit on the left hand.

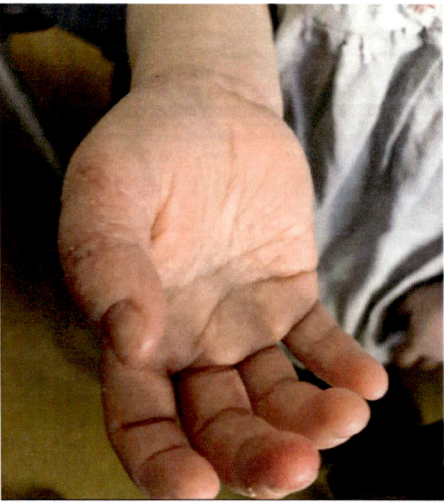

Figure 3. Photograph at pediatric dermatology follow-up 8 days after the initial emergency department visit showing desquamation at the sites of previous bullae and scaly plaques on the distal fingers consistent with her atopic dermatitis.

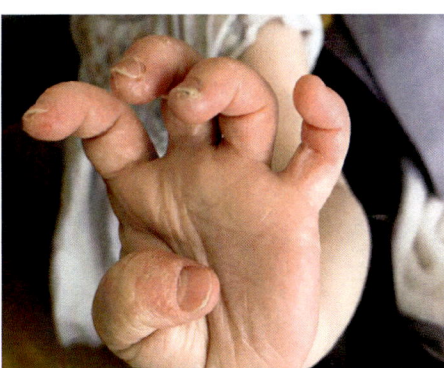

Figure 4. Photograph at pediatric dermatology follow-up 8 days after the initial emergency department visit showing desquamation at the sites of previous bullae and scaly plaques on the distal fingers consistent with her atopic dermatitis.

oral cephalexin to treat a presumed soft tissue infection. The culture was positive for group A *Streptococcus* and methicillin-sensitive *S aureus*. Six days later she had follow-up in the dermatology clinic. Her antibiotic therapy was extended for an additional 5 days given the initial improvement (Figs 3 and 4). It is believed that her underlying atopic dermatitis flare made her more susceptible to a skin infection. Her mom's recent group A streptococcal pharyngitis was thought to be a potential source of infection.

Summary

- Blistering distal dactylitis is a superficial infection of the finger pad of digits, frequently presenting with overlying purulent bullae. It is primarily a clinical diagnosis.

- It is most commonly caused by *Streptococcus* or *Staphylococcus*. (1)(2)(3)

- Systemic antibiotic courses of 7 to 14 days and wound care are the staples for treatment. (1)(2)(3)

- Patients with systemic signs of illness, although rare, would require hospitalization for intravenous antibiotic administration. (15)

References for this article can be found at
https://doi.org/10.1542/pir.2020-004908.

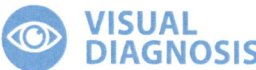

VISUAL
DIAGNOSIS

Skin Lesions on Sensitive Sites: Mimickers of Sexual Abuse in Children

Rachel E. Reingold, BS,* Mandy A. O'Hara, MD, MPH,†‡ Laura E. Levin, MD‡§

*Albert Einstein College of Medicine, Bronx, NY
†Department of Pediatrics and
§Department of Dermatology, Vagelos College of Physicians and Surgeons, Columbia University Irving Medical Center, New York, NY
‡New York–Presbyterian Hospital, New York, NY

PRESENTATION

An 11-year-old boy with no significant medical history presents to a pediatric dermatology clinic with a chief complaint of bumps on the penis. These lesions have been present for more than a year but are growing in number. His mother reports 1 previous episode in which the bumps became red and tender, but they are otherwise asymptomatic. She reports that there are no known contacts with warts. He has a history of attention-deficit/hyperactivity disorder for which he takes dextroamphetamine-amphetamine, and he has no known allergies. He is a developmentally appropriate, healthy child entering seventh grade. He has no trouble concentrating and no changes in mood, sleep, appetite, elimination, or self-image. He feels safe at home, and his mother has no concern for sexual abuse or household stressors.

On examination he is a well-appearing child with approximately 15 hyperpigmented tan and flesh-toned, 1- to 2-mm, dome-shaped papules on the shaft and base of the penis. The papules are smooth, with no central umbilication or overlying surface change (Fig 1).

Without a parent present, he reports no history of unwanted touching or sexual activity, and he does not know what may have caused the rash. Informed consent is obtained from his mother for shave biopsy, and child advocacy is consulted for further input. Results of the biopsy confirm the diagnosis.

DIAGNOSIS

The differential diagnosis for papules on the penis in a child includes, but is not limited to, genital warts, molluscum contagiosum, lichen nitidus, Fordyce spots, and penile syringomas. Cutaneous lesions in the anogenital region may be from infectious, inflammatory, neoplastic, autoimmune, or traumatic etiologies and should be analyzed through a wide lens. (1)(2)(3) Based on the appearance and location of the lesions, a diagnosis of genital warts was favored, and, therefore, the possibility of sexual abuse was raised. Histopathologic analysis of a shave biopsy sample showed dilated ductal structures filled with amorphous material and lined with cuboidal epithelial cells consistent with a syringoma, a benign sweat gland neoplasm.

AUTHOR DISCLOSURE Dr O'Hara's current affiliation is Department of Pediatrics, Einstein School of Medicine, Children's Hospital at Montefiore, Bronx, NY. Ms Reingold and Drs O'Hara and Levin have disclosed no financial relationships relevant to this article. This commentary does not contain a discussion of an unapproved/investigative use of a commercial product/device.

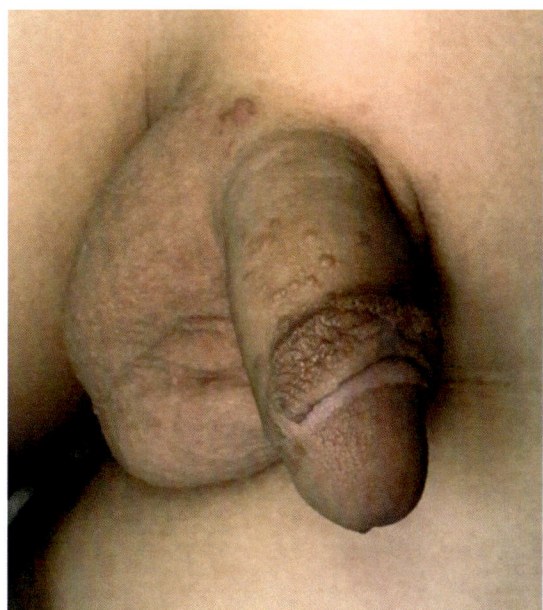

Figure 1. Dome-shaped papules on the shaft and base of the penis.

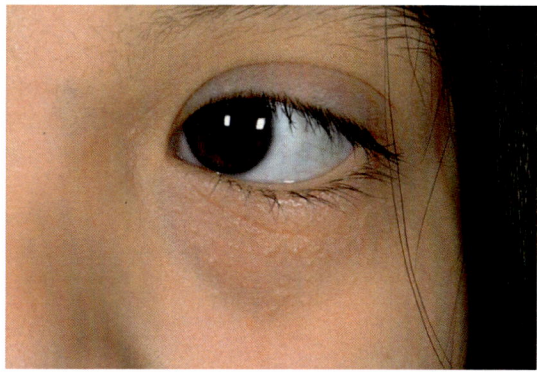

Figure 2. Periorbital syringomas in a female with Down syndrome. (Reprinted with permission from Paller AS, Mancini AJ. Cutaneous tumors and tumor syndromes. In: Paller AS, Mancini AJ, eds. *Hurwitz's Clinical Pediatric Dermatology: A Textbook of Skin Disorders of Childhood and Adolescence.* 5th ed. Amsterdam, the Netherlands: Elsevier; 2015:193–229.) (7)

DISCUSSION

The Condition

Syringomas are benign proliferations of the intraepidermal portion of eccrine sweat ducts. (4) They present as asymptomatic, 1- to 7-mm, smooth, dome-shaped papules that are generally flesh-toned but can be pink, red, tan, or brown. (5) Syringomas occur more often in females than in males and are usually first noted in adolescence and less commonly in childhood. (6) Syringomas are categorized as localized, eruptive, familial, or associated with Down syndrome. (5) Localized syringomas are the predominant subtype and are often periorbital (Fig 2). Other common locations include the cheeks, neck, axilla, trunk, and vulva. (6)(8)(9) Penile syringomas are rare and can present in those younger than 20 years with concern for a sexually transmitted infection (STI) or possible sexual abuse. (8)(9)(10)(11) Detection of distinct histopathologic features, such as proliferation of eccrine ducts, assists in diagnosis.

Treatment and Management

Syringomas are asymptomatic and benign; therefore, active nonintervention with periodic monitoring is a reasonable option, especially in the pediatric setting. (10) Treatment is often cosmetic and depends on factors such as anatomical location, quantity, and patient age. Treatment options include topical retinoids, topical atropine, oral tranilast, and intradermal botulinum toxin A; however, these treatments are limited to case reports. (12)(13)(14)(15) Surgical excision, carbon dioxide laser treatment, and other destructive modalities have been inconsistently effective. (16) Without treatment, syringomas are expected to persist.

Mimickers of Child Sexual Abuse

The differential diagnosis including genital warts led to a concern for possible sexual abuse. Genital warts are caused by human papillomavirus, most commonly types 6 and 11, and present as skin-colored to brown verrucous papules in the genital and perianal areas. (17) In children younger than 3 years, genital warts are more likely to be due to perinatal transmission or benign contact with an infected caregiver. However, in children older than 3 years, there is a greater risk of transmission from autoinoculation and sexual abuse. The American Academy of Pediatrics Committee on Child Abuse and Neglect considers genital warts in infants and prepubertal children suspicious but nondiagnostic for sexual abuse and recommends reporting if a nonsexual source cannot be identified. (18) Molluscum contagiosum, caused by a poxvirus, presents as skin-colored or pink papules with central umbilication and commonly affects school-age or immunocompromised children. (19) Although transmission of molluscum present on the genitalia is possible through sexual contact, transmission is most commonly from autoinoculation and fomites.

Ultimately, in our patient, a comprehensive history that included speaking with the child alone, clinical evaluation with a full physical examination, biopsy, and the help of an interdisciplinary team enabled confirmation of a sweat gland neoplasm and determination of low risk of sexual abuse. This case highlights that anogenital lesions can be difficult to distinguish from STIs and may be mistaken as a sign of sexual abuse, a suspicion that should remain on the differential diagnosis until proved otherwise.

Although the following diagnoses are not in the differential diagnosis for the morphology of the present case, they represent conditions that occur in the anogenital region in children and may similarly be mistaken for child sexual abuse.

Lichen Sclerosus et Atrophicus. Lichen sclerosus et atrophicus (LS&A) is an inflammatory skin condition that commonly affects the anogenital region. It occurs at any age but generally presents in postmenopausal women and prepubertal children with pruritus or purpura on the vulva and possible secondary skin trauma, constipation, or dysuria. (20) Skin findings typically begin as porcelain-white macules or papules that coalesce into the characteristic "figure-of-eight" pattern surrounding the vulvar and perianal regions (Fig 3). Inflammation of the vulvar mucosa leads to atrophy, fragility,

fissuring, telangiectasias, purpura, and scarring with obliteration of normal genital architecture. (22) In males, the characteristic porcelain-white–like sclerotic skin affects the glans, foreskin, and prepuce of the penis, causing phimosis and possible urethral stricture. (23)

LS&A's constellation of skin findings and associated symptoms may raise suspicion for sexual abuse. (3)(24)(25) Although the diagnosis of LS&A is largely clinical, a biopsy can aid in definitive diagnosis. (26) However, even if LS&A is diagnosed, it does not exclude the possibility of sexual abuse. (25)(27)

Crohn Disease. Crohn disease (CD) is characterized by chronic transmural inflammation of the gastrointestinal (GI) tract affecting any mucosal surface from the mouth to the anus. Clinical presentation includes episodic diarrhea, chronic abdominal pain, hematochezia, fatigue, and weight loss. (28) Cutaneous CD describes granulomatous inflammation of the skin and can present with perianal lesions, including skin tags (Fig 4), fissures, anorectal fistulae, scarring, perianal thickening, and ulcers. (30)(31)(32)(33) Approximately two-thirds of cutaneous CD in children involves the genitals, including fissures, edema, swelling, skin tags, abscesses, ulcers, or erythema of the vulva, penis, or perineum. (34) Cutaneous lesions in the perianal and genital regions commonly predate the onset of GI symptoms in children, which can raise suspicion for STIs, trauma, or sexual abuse. (31)(34)(35) In addition to anogenital lesions, CD may present with abdominal pain, a symptom commonly associated with child abuse. (36) Biopsy and additional laboratory data such as liver and pancreatic enzyme levels may be useful tools for diagnosis.

Behçet Disease. Behçet disease (BD) is a rare systemic vasculitis that classically presents with recurrent episodes of uveitis and oral and/or genital ulcers that spontaneously

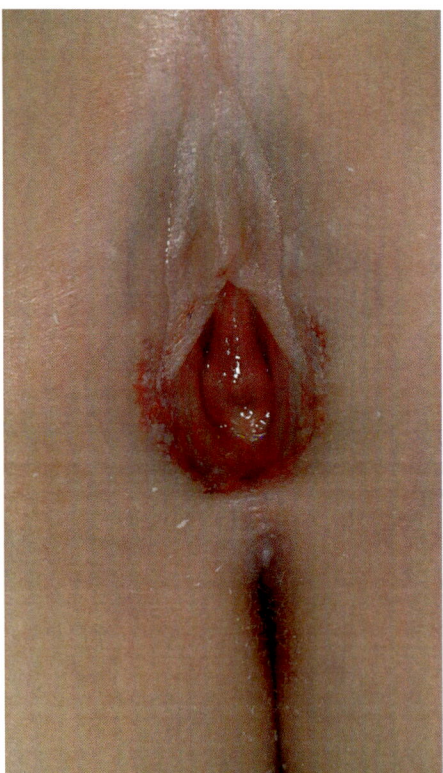

Figure 3. Lichen sclerosus et atrophicus of the labia. Note the porcelain-white atrophy of the labia with purpuric ring surrounding the introitus representative of the condition. (Reprinted with permission from Paller AS, Mancini AJ. Collagen vascular disorders. In: Paller AS, Mancini AJ, eds. *Hurwitz's Clinical Pediatric Dermatology: A Textbook of Skin Disorders of Childhood and Adolescence.* 5th ed. Amsterdam, the Netherlands: Elsevier; 2015:509–539.) (21)

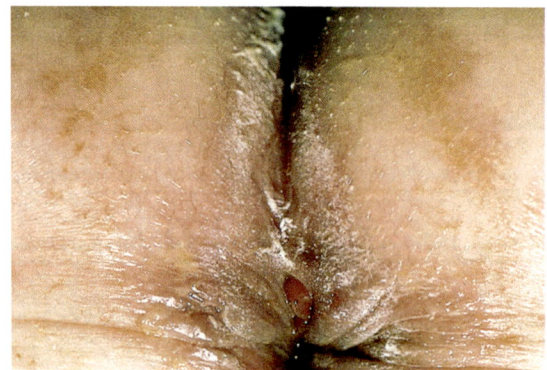

Figure 4. Perianal skin tags of Crohn disease. (Reprinted with permission from Paller AS, Mancini AJ. Skin signs of other systemic diseases. In: Paller AS, Mancini AJ, eds. *Hurwitz's Clinical Pediatric Dermatology: A Textbook of Skin Disorders of Childhood and Adolescence.* 5th ed. Amsterdam, the Netherlands: Elsevier; 2015:573–591.) (29)

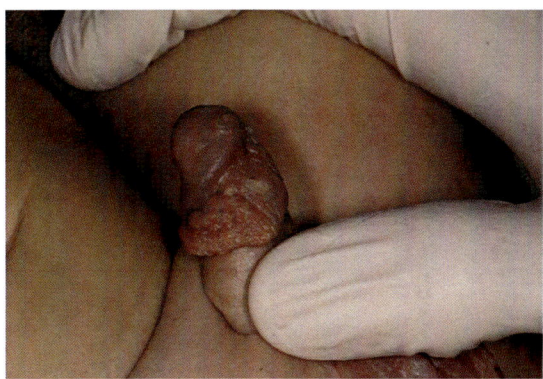

Figure 5. Genital ulcers on the glans penis and foreskin from Behçet disease. (Reprinted with permission from Paller AS, Mancini AJ. Skin signs of other systemic diseases. In: Paller AS, Mancini AJ, eds. *Hurwitz's Clinical Pediatric Dermatology: A Textbook of Skin Disorders of Childhood and Adolescence.* 5th ed. Amsterdam, the Netherlands: Elsevier; 2015:573–591.) (29)

resolve. (37) Inflammation can affect the skin, GI tract, musculoskeletal system, and more. (38) BD generally presents in the second and third decades of life, but it can occur in children. The most common symptoms are oral and genital ulcers, occurring in 97% and 60% to 90% of people, respectively, with 80% having oral ulcers as the presenting symptom. (39) In males, ulcers arise on the scrotum, and in females, on the vulva; however, they can be found in other anogenital regions as well (Fig 5). (37)

Diagnosis may take years due to the fact that there are no unique laboratory or pathological findings. (38) In addition, symptoms may mimic sexually transmitted diseases, vitamin deficiencies, and inflammatory bowel disease, leading a physician down various paths of diagnostic evaluation.

It is important to note that only 4% of sexual abuse referrals have physical findings, with most having normal or nonspecific genital findings. (40)(41) Secondary signs and symptoms of abuse include dysuria or enuresis, genital or anal pain, or acute behavioral changes such as sexualized behavior that in the right clinical context may support the suspicion of abuse. In the case of child disclosure or strong suspicion of abuse, a child abuse pediatric specialist can assist by performing STI testing and a colposcope evaluation of the genital and anal anatomy to rule out additional findings concerning for abuse.

Referral to a pediatric dermatologist in the evaluation of anogenital cutaneous lesions may help to diagnose a dermatologic condition. This is not to suggest that by making a medical diagnosis, sexual abuse can be effectively omitted from speculation. Rather, it is to highlight that there exist diagnoses that imitate sexual abuse and should be considered by an interdisciplinary team.

Patient Course

Active nonintervention with periodic monitoring was recommended. This decision was made with the pediatrician after discussion that the biopsy results and history eliminated above average concern for sexual abuse. There was no further indication for a child advocacy evaluation.

SUMMARY

- In the case of cutaneous lesions in the anogenital region suspicious for child sexual abuse, partnership with an interdisciplinary team, including a pediatric dermatologist and a child abuse pediatric specialist, may aid in diagnosis and help to avoid unnecessary evaluation or mandated reporting when no additional signs or concern for sexual abuse are suspected.

- Dermatologic conditions and sexual abuse can present together and are not mutually exclusive. Herein, although the diagnosis of penile syringomas was determined, it was the medical interview and consultation with child abuse pediatric specialists that helped to effectively rule out sexual abuse.

- Dermatologic conditions that manifest in the anogenital area in children may be difficult to distinguish from child sexual abuse.

References for this article can be found at https://doi.org/10.1542/pir.2020-004317.

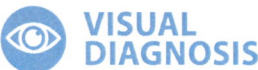 **VISUAL DIAGNOSIS**

Sudden-Onset Black Facial Lesions in an 11-year-old Boy

Catherine Burger, MD*

*Vanderbilt University Medical Center, Nashville, TN

PRESENTATION

An 11-year-old boy presents to the emergency department with a chief complaint of rash. He noticed 2 dark areas of discoloration to the right side of his face this morning when looking in the mirror. The dark areas do not hurt but are slightly itchy. He lives in Tennessee and went swimming in a local lake with family one day before his emergency department visit but did not notice any bites, new exposures, or trauma to the area. He has never had a rash like this before. No other family members feel ill or have a rash. He has not had a fever or any recent illness. He has no known medical history, does not take any medications, and has never had surgery. He is up to date on immunizations.

Vital signs were within normal limits. On examination the patient has 2 non-palpable, nontender, well-demarcated, black macules to the right cheek, approximately 7 mm and 4 mm in diameter, with 2 to 3 cm of surrounding mild erythema without sloughing or blistering. No other lesions on skin evaluation. He is well-appearing and has no other abnormal HEENT findings on examination. His cardiopulmonary, abdominal, and neurologic examination findings are normal as well.

Given his well appearance, lack of other symptoms, and reassuring vital signs, his initial evaluation included consultation with a dermatologist, which revealed the diagnosis.

DIAGNOSIS

This patient has black spot poison ivy from a toxicodendron exposure.

DISCUSSION

The differential diagnosis for new, focal, well-demarcated skin discoloration includes traumatic injury, malignancy, vasculitis, allergic reaction, drug reaction, and infection. In this case the sudden onset of skin discoloration makes melanoma or congenital focal skin discoloration less likely. His well appearance and lack of fever or systemic symptoms is also reassuring against endocarditis with septic emboli or other serious bacterial infections. Purpura, or skin discoloration due to disruption of small blood vessels as seen in vasculitis, is often raised and palpable, unlike the patient's macules in this case. In addition, vasculitis often presents with systemic symptoms such as arthritis or abdominal pain, which were also absent in this case. For black spot poison ivy, the skin discoloration should be nontender and the borders should be well-demarcated, unlike that of a bruise or scattered petechia from

AUTHOR DISCLOSURE Dr Burger has disclosed no financial relationships relevant to this article. This manuscript does not contain a discussion of an unapproved/investigative use of a commercial product/device.

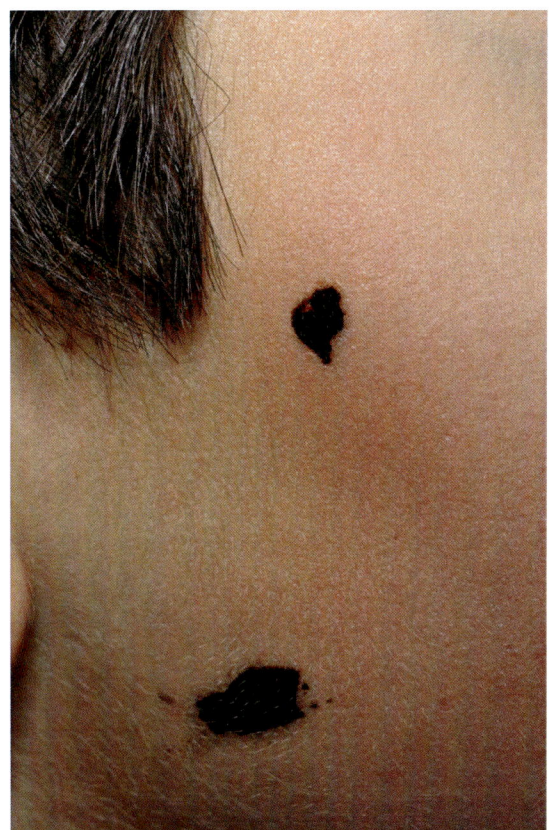

Figure. Nonpalpable, nontender macules on the patient's right cheek on the day of the emergency department visit.

in high enough concentrations on exposure to cause the black lacquer. (2)

The black lacquer can develop on any solid surface, such as clothing or tools, and can be seen on previously injured parts of the plant. The resin is thought to seal the injury and protect the plant. For many centuries, sap from Japanese lacquer trees, a closely related plant, has been used to produce a black surface on furniture. Contact with the furniture years after production has been found to cause allergic contact dermatitis. (3)

Although severe cases of black spot poison ivy can cause epidermal necrosis, the condition is not dangerous and does not leave a scar. (4) No treatment is needed for removal of the black lacquer; it is self-limited. Patients and families with black spot poison ivy should be counseled on the potential for development of allergic contact dermatitis and the expected resolution of discoloration in 1 to 2 weeks.

PATIENT COURSE

This patient followed up with his pediatrician 3 weeks later and noted no further skin discoloration or symptoms.

Summary

- Diagnosis of black spot poison ivy is based on a detailed history and physical examination.

- On initial presentation, patients with black spot poison ivy should have no further signs or symptoms beyond the sudden-onset, well-demarcated black skin discoloration and mild local irritant dermatitis.

- The black skin discoloration is a result of exposure to a toxicodendron plant and contact with an oily resin that is released in high concentration when the plant is injured. The resin is initially clear and then oxidizes to a black color over minutes to hours.

- Patients with black spot poison ivy should be counseled on the potential for development of allergic contact dermatitis and the expected resolution of discoloration in 1 to 2 weeks without permanent damage.

Acknowledgments
Thank you to Dr Larry Stack for his review of the manuscript and for obtaining the photograph.

References for this article can be found at
https://doi.org/10.1542/pir.2020-001834.

trauma. Lack of additional symptoms and no recent medications make drug reaction less likely as well. On initial presentation, patients with black spot poison ivy should have no further signs or symptoms beyond the black skin discoloration and mild local irritant dermatitis.

Black spot poison ivy is an uncommon emergency department presentation after exposure to a toxicodendron plant such as poison ivy or poison oak. It is the result of contact with an oily resin that is released in high concentration when the plant is injured. (1) The resin deposits in the superficial layers of the skin, the stratum corneum and epidermis. The resin is initially not easily visible, but within minutes to hours oxidation causes the formation of a black lacquer. The discoloration cannot be pealed or cleaned off and often is present for 1 to 2 weeks.

A surrounding irritant dermatitis is often present on the day of exposure, causing local, mild erythema. Contact allergic dermatitis may then develop days to weeks later in sensitized individuals. The same oily resin that causes the black lacquer is also responsible for the commonly seen allergic contact dermatitis; however, it is not often present

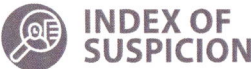

INDEX OF SUSPICION

Lumbar Skin Lesion in a Term Infant

Shannon E. Brockman, MD,[*,†] Katherine M. Ottolini, MD,[†‡] Elizabeth V. Schulz, MD[†‡]

[*]United States Navy Medicine Readiness and Training Command Okinawa, Okinawa, Japan

[†]Department of Pediatrics, F. Edward Hebert School of Medicine, Uniformed Services University, Bethesda, MD

[‡]Department of Neonatology, 18th Healthcare Operations Squadron, Kadena AB, Okinawa, Japan

PRESENTATION

A newborn girl is noted to have a midline lumbar depression at birth. She is twin A born by uncomplicated vaginal delivery at 38 weeks and 5 days of gestation to a 31-year-old gravida 2, now para 3 mother after dichorionic/diamniotic twin pregnancy via in vitro fertilization. The pregnancy was otherwise complicated by diet-controlled gestational diabetes and maternal history of herpes simplex virus without lesions or prodromal symptoms at the time of delivery. Maternal medications during pregnancy included prenatal vitamins and valacyclovir prophylaxis. The infant transitions well and requires only routine care at the time of delivery.

Her initial physical examination reveals a circumferential 1 × 0.5-cm punched-out, skin-covered lesion overlying the midline spine at the level of L4-L5 vertebrae with surrounding dermal melanocytosis extending from the midline to the left flank (Fig 1). The examination findings are otherwise normal, with appropriate tone for age, symmetrical movement of all extremities, and intact neonatal reflexes. Spinal ultrasonography is performed on the second day after birth because of the cutaneous findings and is notable for a low-lying spinal cord with conus termination at the level of L3-L4 with a thickened appearance of the filum terminale. Head ultrasonography is also performed, and findings are normal.

DISCUSSION

Differential Diagnosis

The differential diagnosis of a punched-out skin lesion overlying the lumbar region includes, but is not limited to, a lumbosacral dimple, vascular malformation, skin atrophy, cutis aplasia, dermal sinus, and ulcerative or necrotizing skin infection. A sacral dimple is a depression in the skin of the lower back, typically occurring just above the crease between the buttocks. Lumbosacral dimples are common in newborn infants and are usually normal anatomic variants when solitary and located entirely in the gluteal cleft. However, the presence of multiple dimples, dimples with a diameter greater than 5 mm or located greater than 2.5 cm above the anus, or those associated with other cutaneous abnormalities warrant further evaluation for underlying occult spinal dysraphism (OSD). (1) Vascular malformations, including port-wine stains and hemangiomas, vary from simple macules to complex structures involving multiple layers of skin and subcutaneous tissue. They can be composed of arteries, veins, capillaries, and/or lymphatic vessels and may be markers of OSD when overlying the spine. Skin

AUTHOR DISCLOSURE Drs Brockman, Ottolini, and Schulz have disclosed no financial relationships relevant to this article. This commentary does not contain a discussion of an unapproved/investigative use of a commercial product/device.

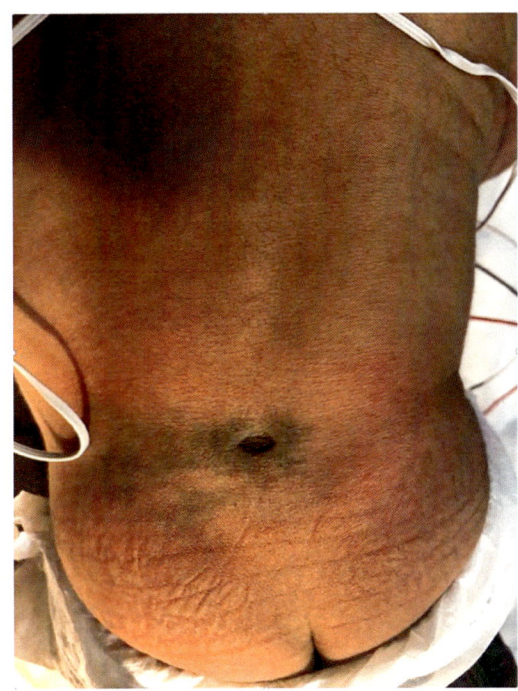

Figure 1. Photograph demonstrating a punched-out lesion with a melanocytic area overlying lumbar and sacral region skin. This photograph has not been enhanced or altered in any way.

atrophy is characterized by thinning of the epidermis, dermis, and underlying subcutaneous tissue. Cutis aplasia, or aplasia cutis congenita (ACC), is the congenital absence of skin, which can appear ulcerated or scarred at birth. (2) Primarily a clinical diagnosis, cutis aplasia overlying the lumbosacral spine has also been associated with OSD. (2)

A dermal sinus is a midline epithelium-lined tract from the skin to the cranial or spinal cavity caused by incomplete neural tube closure. Dermal sinuses predispose the infant to serious infections, including bacterial meningitis and intraspinal abscesses. (1)(3) Necrotizing soft tissue infections are characterized by the destruction of the skin and underlying soft tissues and can involve the epidermis, dermis, subcutaneous tissue, fascia, and muscle. In neonates, necrotizing infections most typically occur in the abdominal or perineal area as omphalitis, balanitis after circumcision, or surgical site infection after hernia repair. (4)

Term infants with midline cutaneous lesions overlying the spine, including elevated lesions (eg, tissue appendages, masses, hair patches), cutis aplasia, hemangiomas, or atypical sacral dimples, require neuroimaging with spinal ultrasonography and/or magnetic resonance imaging (MRI) to ensure early detection of underlying spinal

dysraphism. (5) Due to concern for underlying OSD, our patient underwent a nonsedated MRI of the head and lumbar spine. Although notable for suboptimal quality due to low image resolution and significant motion artifact, the MRI demonstrated a low-lying conus medullaris without clear visualization of the filum terminale. The diagnosis of cutis aplasia with an underlying tethered spinal cord is made based on physical examination and neuroimaging.

The Condition

First reported in the mid-18th century, cutis aplasia, also known as ACC, is a dermal examination finding that can be seen in isolation (incidence 1:3,000) or in conjunction with various trisomies or syndromes. (6)(7) Patients with ACC are classified into 1 of 9 groups based on the location and configuration of the skin defect, presence of associated abnormalities, and mode of inheritance. This classification system has recently been updated to include specific molecular-genetic diagnoses associated with some lesions. (2)(8) Patients with ACC have a 20% mortality rate, although this is likely secondary to associated underlying syndromes rather than the cutaneous lesion itself. (9)(10) Sex distribution is equivalent and familial cases have been reported, although no singular underlying cause has been identified. (11) Most lesions are small (<3 cm in diameter) but have been reported up to 7.5 cm. (12)(13) The lesion is typically a well-circumscribed area with absence or thinning of the epidermis and underlying dermal atrophy on histologic examination. (12) Most cases of cutis aplasia occur on the scalp (~80%–85%) and extremities; alternative locations include the anterior chest wall and trunk. (2) A ring of dark, coarse hair may surround the cutaneous lesion, known as "hair collar sign." (14)

Cutis aplasia of the scalp may be associated with aplasia of the skull itself as well as a sagittal or dural sinus hemorrhage. (12) Although isolated cutis aplasia in the lumbosacral region is a well-recognized neurocutaneous marker for OSD, our literature review revealed only 1 case report and 1 textbook photograph of this rare, but important, physical examination finding. (15)(16)

ACC has also been noted in surviving infants of multiple-gestation pregnancies complicated by fetus papyraceus, a phenomenon of fetal mummification after intrauterine death. In these cases, the questionable area can appear in a stellate, rather than a circumferential, shape and usually appears on the trunk. (17) Interestingly, fetus papyraceus has been increasingly seen in the era of assisted reproductive technology and a higher incidence of multiple-gestation pregnancies, leading to a proposed increased risk of cutis aplasia in this specific population. However, up to 95% of the reported fetus papyraceus cases are seen in monochorionic twin pregnancies with a first-trimester fetal demise, and our case was the product of a dichorionic/diamniotic twin pregnancy. In addition, the lesion in our patient was the traditional circumferential shape versus the alternative stellate pattern commonly seen in fetus papyraceus. (17) The fetus papyraceus lesion can have a similar appearance as skin atrophy, although the history of the twin gestation will be foretelling.

Treatment and Management

Cutis Aplasia. The treatment of cutis aplasia is focused primarily on management of the cutaneous defect. Small lesions (<3 cm) may not require surgical intervention because the skin typically heals via secondary intention. This is generally the case with parchment paper–like lesions, which have the appearance of thinning tissue with a crinkled or scarlike external layer. Wound care of granulomatous-appearing lesions includes local infection precautions to allow epithelialization of the lesion, which may take weeks to months. Commercial wound care products may decrease healing time. More extensive lesions (≥4 cm) may require the involvement of dermatology and plastic surgery for tissue expansion and skin grafts or flaps depending on the breadth of the area involved and surgeon evaluation/preference. (18) Lesions over bony prominences at risk for prolonged pressure in primarily supine-

positioned infants carry a substantial risk of infectious and hemorrhagic complications, and these lesions may require early surgical intervention. (7)(19)

Tethered Cord. Cutaneous markers concerning for OSD, including cutis aplasia, should prompt medical care teams to perform neuroimaging studies. If a tethered cord is identified on MRI, management varies based on the child's age at diagnosis. For patients presenting with neurologic symptoms such as pain or loss of bladder or bowel control, timely repair is indicated to preserve neurologic function. The decision to perform the untethering is controversial in asymptomatic patients and requires a risk/benefit analysis because the procedure does not consistently result in improved neurologic outcomes and carries a risk of subsequent retethering. (20) All children with a tethered cord warrant ongoing evaluation by both their primary care provider and subspecialty teams through adolescence to monitor for neurologic dysfunction and orthopedic abnormalities.

Case Progression

Due to clinical suspicion, the infant was transferred to a pediatric subspecialty center to undergo MRI at 3 months of age. The repeated MRI confirmed a low-lying conus medullaris terminating at the mid-L3 vertebral body with a rightward deviation of the most inferior aspect (Fig 2). After diagnostic evaluation by pediatric neurosurgery, the infant underwent an uncomplicated tethered cord release and excision of the overlying cutis aplasia at 6 months of age. After surgery she remained at the tertiary care center for 2 weeks to facilitate immediate postoperative management

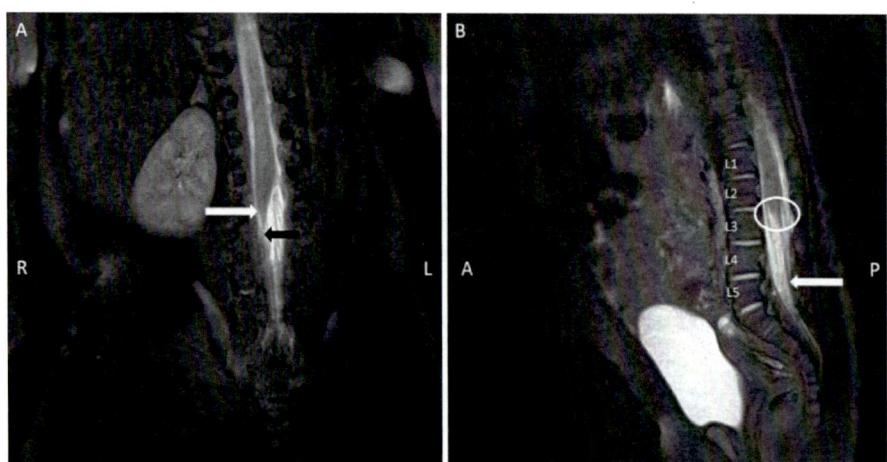

Figure 2. Magnetic resonance imaging findings. A. Coronal T2-weighted image demonstrates rightward deviation of the spinal cord, specifically the conus medullaris (white arrow) and filum terminale (black arrow). B. Sagittal T2-weighted image demonstrates low-lying conus (circle), typically defined as a conus medullaris distal to the patient's L2 vertebra, and posterior (P) tethering of the distal cord (arrow) with a comparatively thickened filum.

and recovery. After discharge she continues monthly home-based early intervention monitoring with physical therapy for gross motor development follow-up. She is progressing well, with no current neurodevelopmental impairments. Owing to the risk of retethering, follow-up with the neurosurgeon may be required if she demonstrates any new signs of neurologic deterioration, including gait abnormality, muscle atrophy, bowel or bladder dysfunction, lumbosacral pain, foot deformities, or scoliosis.

Lessons for the Clinician

- Head ultrasonography, spinal ultrasonography, and/or magnetic resonance imaging are first-line neuroimaging studies when cutis aplasia is present on the scalp or back to evaluate for underlying abnormalities of the brain, spine, or bone (skull and vertebrae).
- Cutis aplasia involving small cutaneous defects (<3 cm) may be managed with supportive care while awaiting skin reepithelialization, whereas larger lesions (≥4 cm) or those overlying bony prominences may require surgical intervention with skin grafting.
- Early symptoms of neurologic dysfunction associated with tethered cord include bowel and bladder dysfunction and delayed motor milestones (ie, walking), although most often infants are asymptomatic, with a more insidious onset later in life.

References for this article can be found at https://doi.org/10.1542/pir.2020-001834.

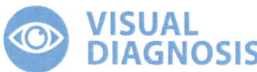

VISUAL DIAGNOSIS

An Ulcerating Perineal Rash in an 8-month-old Girl

Nisha Ganesh, MD,* Rena Kasick, MD,*† Emily Graham, MD*†‡

*The Ohio State University College of Medicine, Columbus, OH
†Nationwide Children's Hospital, Columbus, OH
‡The Ohio State University Wexner Medical Center, Columbus, OH

PRESENTATION

A previously healthy 8-month-old female presents to the emergency department (ED) with diarrhea and an unusual diaper rash. Her symptoms began 6 days prior with fever and congestion. She was initially diagnosed with a viral upper respiratory infection and bilateral otitis media and was prescribed cephalexin by her primary care physician. Two days later, she developed diarrhea and a painful diaper rash. Cephalexin was changed to cefdinir due to concern for antibiotic-induced diarrhea. After 5 days of treatment, antibiotics were discontinued. Before this presentation to the ED, she had been evaluated multiple times in the ED for worsening diaper rash and was prescribed a barrier cream, topical anti-fungal cream, and mupirocin ointment without improvement. Her medical history includes 1 prior episode of acute otitis media. Her immunizations are up to date. She takes no medications. She lives at home with her mother and father. There have been no known sick contacts, no recent travel, no known insect bites, and no animal exposures aside from the family's pet dog.

Her vital signs on presentation are as follows: temperature, 98.6°F (37°C); heart rate, 160 beats/min; respiratory rate, 40 breaths/min; blood pressure, 100/48 mm Hg; oxygen saturation, 95% on room air. Her parents report that she has had profuse watery diarrhea and decreased urine output, and they describe her behavior as fussy and irritable. Her review of systems is negative for vomiting, blood in the stool, abdominal pain or distension, easy bleeding or bruising, weight loss or inadequate weight gain, recurrent infections, and rashes aside from the current diaper rash. On physical examination, she has multiple large areas of ulceration and necrosis surrounded by halos of erythema in the genitourinary region (Fig 1). Her laboratory studies are significant for blood urea nitrogen of 24 mg/dL (8.6 mmol/L), creatinine of 0.73 mg/dL (55.7 μmol/L), hemoglobin of 9.1 g/dL (91 g/L), platelet count of $93 \times 10^3/\mu L$ ($93 \times 10^9/L$), and an absolute neutrophil count of 1,220/μL ($1.22 \times 10^9/L$). Based on the clinical appearance of the rash and results of subsequent bacterial wound cultures, a diagnosis is made.

DIAGNOSIS

The appearance of this patient's ulcerative perineal rash is consistent with ecthyma gangrenosum (EG). Her blood cultures remained negative; however, her bacterial wound cultures returned with growth of *Pseudomonas aeruginosa*, confirming the diagnosis of EG.

AUTHOR DISCLOSURE Drs. Ganesh, Graham, and Kasick have disclosed no financial relationships relevant to this article. This commentary does not contain a discussion of an unapproved/investigative use of a commercial product/device.

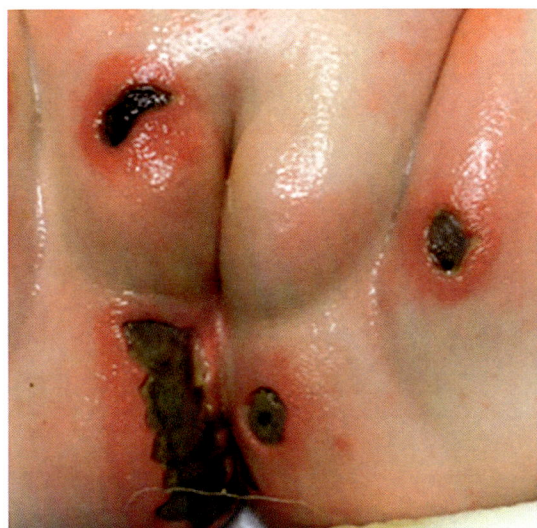
Figure 1. Perineal skin lesions in a previously healthy 8-month-old female on hospital presentation.

DISCUSSION

Clinical Presentation and Pathogenesis

EG is an ulcerating and necrotizing skin infection classically associated with *P aeruginosa* bacteremia in immunocompromised patients. These lesions typically begin as erythematous macules or papules that subsequently evolve into pustular or bullous lesions and finally necrotic ulcers surrounded by a halo of erythema. (1) Lesions most commonly occur in the anogenital area in 57% of cases. Other areas of involvement include the extremities in 30%, trunk in 6%, and face in 6% of cases. (1)

EG generally results from bacteremia with hematologic dissemination to the skin and soft tissue, but may also present as a primary skin infection. (1) These cutaneous lesions form secondary to ischemic necrosis, which follows bacterial invasion and toxin mediated destruction of arterial media and adventitia. (2)

Differential Diagnosis

Although typically caused by *P aeruginosa*, the microbial differential diagnosis is broad and includes gram-positive bacteria (*Staphylococcus aureus*, *Streptococcus pyogenes*), other gram-negative bacteria (*Aeromonas hydrophila*, *Klebsiella pneumonia*, *Serratia marcescens*, *Xanthomonas maltophilia*, *Morganella morganii*, *Escherichia coli*, *Citrobacter freundii*, *Corynebacterium diphtheriae*, *Neisseria gonorrhea*), fungi (*Candida albicans*, *Aspergillus fumigatus*), mucormycosis, and herpes simplex virus. (3)(4) These microbes

may form identical lesions; therefore, blood and wound cultures are necessary for an accurate diagnosis.

Other conditions that may mimic EG include pyoderma gangrenosum (PG), recluse spider bites, cutaneous vasculitis, and cutaneous anthrax. Like EG, PG can present as an expanding nodule that ulcerates and becomes necrotic. However, PG is typically painful at the site of ulceration and may exhibit pathergy, the development of ulcerative skin lesions at sites of minor trauma. Patients may also have symptoms or history of associated underlying systemic disease such as inflammatory bowel disease. Ultimately, tissue biopsy and culture can distinguish between the 2. (5) Recluse spider bites also mimic EG, but present with a single, flat lesion that is smaller than 10 cm and has a pale center. Unlike EG, the lesions of a recluse spider bite typically do not swell, produce pus, or ulcerate sooner than 7 days from presentation. These signs are more indicative of an infectious process. (6) Necrotic ulcers may also be found in cutaneous vasculitis. These lesions are likely to occur symmetrically in the lower extremities and dependent areas or in areas corresponding to constrictive clothing. Patients may have other symptoms of a connective tissue disease or recent introduction of a new medication. If suspicion of vasculitis is high, skin biopsy is the most reliable method of diagnosis. (7) Cutaneous anthrax also presents as a papule that evolves into a necrotic ulcer, but in the absence of bioterrorism, patients have a history of contact with animals or animal hides. (8) Based on clinical and laboratory findings, other considerations in the differential diagnosis of EG may include bullous fixed drug eruption, disseminated intravascular coagulation (purpura fulminans), septic emboli, livedoid vasculopathy, warfarin-induced skin necrosis, heparin-induced thrombocytopenia, and calciphylaxis (skin ischemia and necrosis secondary to calcium deposition in the arterioles and capillaries of the skin and subcutaneous tissue, usually in the setting of end-stage renal disease). (4)

Risk Factors for Disease

The most frequent risk factor for EG is neutropenia in patients with malignancy or patients taking immune modulating agents. (9)(10) EG rarely occurs in otherwise healthy individuals; however, there are case reports of EG in patients without any known classic risk factors on presentation. Many of these patients were subsequently found to have transient risk factors for EG or EG as a first presentation of an underlying disease. In a literature review of 18 previously healthy patients presenting with EG, 9 had neutropenia (7 transient neutropenia, 1 chronic neutropenia, and 1 cyclic neutropenia), 7 had prior antibiotic exposure, 4 had hypogammaglobinemia, 3 had preceding viral infections, 2 had intraabdominal abscess, 2 had preceding severe acute illness, 2 had abnormal neutrophil function, and 1 had preceding diarrhea (many patients had multiple risk factors). (9) Given the possibility of EG as a presentation of a previously undiagnosed immune deficiency, patients without typical risk factors should undergo a comprehensive immunologic evaluation.

Principles of Management

Management of EG includes collection of blood and tissue cultures and empiric antimicrobial therapy followed by directed antimicrobial therapy once culture results are available. Empiric therapy for EG should include an antipseudomonal β-lactam (piperacillin/tazobactam), cephalosporin (cefepime, ceftazidime), carbapenem (meropenem, imipenem), or fluoroquinolone (ciprofloxacin). Aminoglycosides may be added for combination therapy in high risk patients (immunocompromised patients, patients with risk factors for multidrug resistant organisms) or in severe presentations (septic shock). Antibiotic duration is typically 10 to 14 days. (11) Surgical debridement is often required. (4) Wound care recommendations specific to EG were not found in the literature. In our patient, the wound care team was consulted and skin barrier cream followed by petrolatum-based wound dressings were applied.

Prognosis

The mortality rate of *P aeruginosa* sepsis in previously healthy children is estimated at 55% based on a review of the literature. (12) Although much lower, the mortality rate for nonbacteremic EG is still substantial at 7% to 15%. (13)(14) Mortality in these cases was attributed to progression of infection and subsequent sepsis. However, these case series are less generalizable to the pediatric population, as the median age in each case series was 63 and 50 years, respectively, and to our previously healthy patient, as all patients in these case series were immunocompromised, most commonly with hematologic malignancy.

HOSPITAL COURSE

The infectious disease service was consulted, and she was started empirically on piperacillin/tazobactam. Bacterial wound and stool cultures returned positive for *P aeruginosa*. Herpes simplex virus culture was negative. Blood cultures were negative. Other significant findings included a positive nasopharynx rhinovirus polymerase

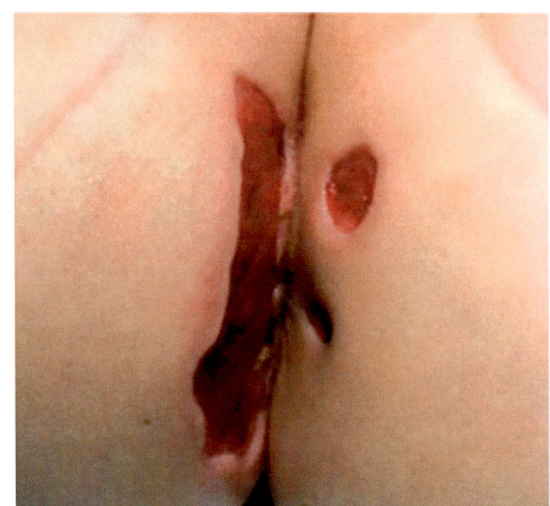

Figure 2. Healing perineal wounds after antibiotics and surgical debridement.

chain reaction and an abdominal ultrasound showing right lower quadrant inflammatory enteritis. Her wounds were surgically debrided, and intraoperative bacterial tissue cultures grew *P aeruginosa* and *Bacteroides fragilis*. Intraoperative fungal cultures were negative. Pathology results demonstrated sections of necrotic skin in which the epidermis was absent, and the dermis and subcutaneous tissue showed extensive coagulative necrosis and patchy acute inflammation. Gram-stain showed rare gram-negative rods within the necrotic tissues. Evaluation for underlying immunodeficiency was negative with normal immunoglobulins, negative human immunodeficiency virus testing, normal oxidative burst assay, and normal T and B lymphocyte immunophenotyping. Her diarrhea resolved and the appearance of her wounds improved. Her acute kidney injury, neutropenia, and thrombocytopenia resolved, but she continued to have mild anemia. She was transitioned to oral ciprofloxacin and metronidazole to complete a 14-day course and recovered uneventfully (Fig 2).

Summary

- EG is a skin infection that appears as necrotic ulcers surrounded by an erythematous halo.

- Although typically associated with *P aeruginosa* bacteremia in immunocompromised patients, EG can occur in previously healthy individuals and may also present as a localized skin infection in the absence of bacteremia.

- Risk factors for EG in otherwise healthy patients include preceding viral infection, recent antibiotic use, and transient neutropenia.

- EG may also be the presenting condition in a patient with an underlying immune deficiency, thus a comprehensive immunologic evaluation should be pursued.

Acknowledgment

This case is based on a presentation by Dr Graham at the Society of Hospital Medicine conference, clinical vignettes poster competition in Orlando, Florida, Poster Session: April 9, 2018, Poster Number: 368.

References for this article can be found at https://doi.org/10.1542/pir.2020-0052.

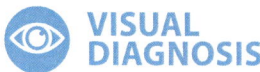

VISUAL DIAGNOSIS

An Unusual Pigmented Plaque in a Newborn

Jena Song, DO, MPH,* Jose Bustillo, DO,* Sherin Meledathu, DO*

*Department of Internal Medicine and Pediatrics, Newark Beth Israel Medical Center and Children's of New Jersey, Newark, NJ

PRESENTATION

A full-term, large for gestational age newborn girl, is born via vaginal delivery to a 32-year-old gravida 3, para 3 mother with a generally uncomplicated pregnancy. The pediatrics team has been called to the delivery for meconium-stained amniotic fluid. The infant does not appear to be in respiratory distress and has Apgar scores of 9 and 9 at 1 and 5 minutes, respectively. Her blood glucose level is 45 mg/dL. Upon inspection, she is noted to have a large, raised, hyperpigmented plaque covering the right side of her head, measuring 18 × 15 cm (Figs 1 and 2). This plaque is accompanied by greater than 20 other macules, patches, and plaques diffusely distributed throughout the body that are either hyper or hypopigmented, have either smooth or irregular borders, and vary in size from 0.5 to 3 cm (Fig 3). The patient also has multiple areas of blue-gray pigmented patches on her sacrum, but no sacral dimple is evident. Her neurologic examination reveals a newborn who is alert, responsive, and has normal primitive reflexes and tone for gestational age. Her head circumference is 35.5 cm (53rd percentile). No dysmorphic features are noted, and the remainder of the examination is remarkable only for a systolic heart murmur.

Our patient is admitted to the NICU for close monitoring and further evaluation of her skin lesions. Initial testing in the NICU includes an ophthalmologic examination, head ultrasound, and magnetic resonance imaging (MRI) of the spine, all of which are normal. The infant also has an MRI of the brain completed, which shows a 2-mm faint T1 hyperintense lesion in the right frontal lobe (Fig 4). Furthermore, an echocardiogram is performed to evaluate a persistent murmur; there is a small to moderate-sized patient ductus arteriosus and a patent foramen ovale. The patient passes her newborn hearing screen bilaterally. The physical examination, in conjunction with the MRI findings, confirms the diagnosis.

DIAGNOSIS

The differential diagnoses for this type of skin lesion in a newborn are vast and include, but are not limited to, the following: Becker nevus, Spitz nevus, epidermal nevus syndrome, nevus sebaceous, plexiform neurofibroma, and Urbach-Wiethe disease (lipoid proteinosis). The descriptions of each of these can be found in Table 1. However, the physical examination of our patient is most consistent with a giant congenital melanocytic nevi (CMN). This, along with the MRI of the brain finding, supports the diagnosis of neurocutaneous melanosis (NCM).

AUTHOR DISCLOSURE Drs Song, Bustillo, and Meledathu have disclosed no financial relationships relevant to this article. This commentary does not contain a discussion of an unapproved/investigative use of a commercial product/device.

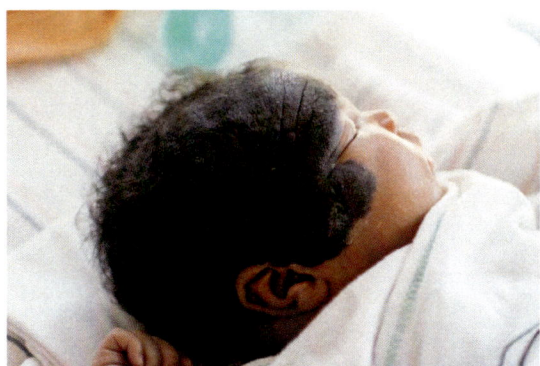

Figure 1. Gross visualization of plaque throughout the body. A large, raised, hyperpigmented plaque, measuring 18 × 15 cm, covering the right side of the infant's scalp. © 2017–2020, Jena Song, DO, MPH. All rights reserved. Reprinted with permission.

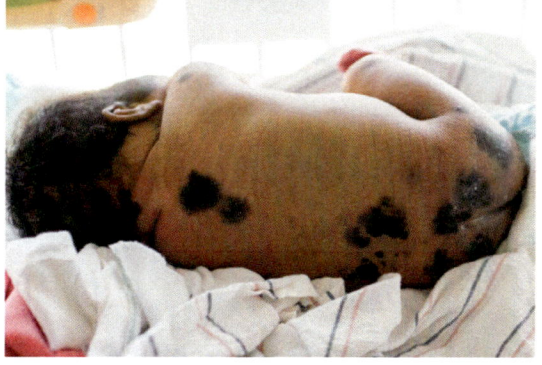

Figure 3. Gross visualization of plaque throughout the body. Numerous hyperpigmented macules, patches, and patches of smaller caliber covering the right shoulder, posterior neck, back, and gluteal regions. © 2017–2020, Jena Song, DO, MPH. All rights reserved. Reprinted with permission.

DISCUSSION

CMN, also known colloquially as moles, are present in approximately 1% to 3% of neonates, making them a common finding. (9) They are typically a benign proliferation of a specific melanocyte, the nevus cell, and are either present at birth or develop within the first few months of life. Multiple authors have attempted to describe CMN by size; Krengel et al (10) have proposed the most recent definitions in 2012. They characterize CMN as small, medium, large, and giant according to the anticipated diameter of the nevus in adulthood. Small and medium lesions range from less than 1.5 to 20 cm in diameter, large CMN are 20 to 40 cm, and giant CMN are greater than 40 cm in adults. (10) Kadonaga and Frieden (11) define large CMN in children as a lesion greater than 9 cm on the head or greater than 6 cm on the body.

Large and giant CMN are less common than small and medium nevi, and occur in roughly 1 in every 20,000 births. (12) It is imperative to recognize large and giant CMN because these lesions are associated with an increased risk of multiple complications. This includes NCM, a neuroectodermal dysplasia. NCM is a rare disease characterized by aberrant proliferation of melanocytes within the central nervous system (CNS) and skin. (13) Symptomatic NCM is estimated to affect 3% to 10% of infants and children with high-risk CMN; this was first described by Rokitanksy in 1861. (14)

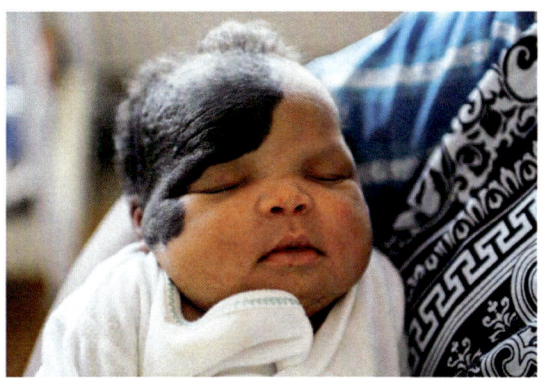

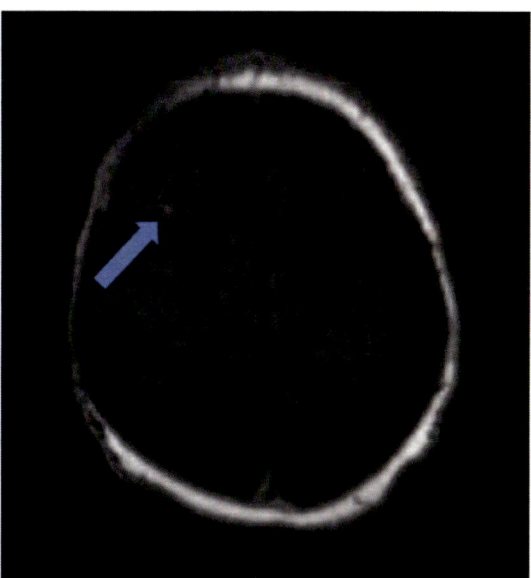

Figure 2. Gross visualization of plaque throughout the body. Further visualization of large, hyperpigmented plaque extending to the right maxillary region and right upper eyelid. © 2017–2020, Jena Song, DO, MPH. All rights reserved. Reprinted with permission.

Figure 4. Magnetic resonance imaging of the brain. A 2-mm faint T1 hyperintense lesion in the right frontal lobe. © 2017–2020, Jena Song, DO, MPH. All rights reserved. Reprinted with permission.

Table 1. Differential Diagnoses for Large/Giant Congenital Melanocytic Nevi

CONDITION	CLINICAL FEATURES
Becker nevus (1)	• Asymptomatic irregular tan-to-brown patch, most commonly located over the shoulder, upper chest, or back • Onset: peripubertal period but can be present at birth
Spitz nevus (2)	• Uncommon melanocytic lesion • Composed of large epithelioid and/or spindled cells • Presents in childhood or adolescence • Sharply circumscribed, dome-shaped, pink-red papule, plaque, or nodule • Most common locations: face or lower extremities • Risk of developing into melanoma
Epidermal nevus syndrome (3)(4)	• Benign, hamartomatous growths of the skin • Subtle, linear patches and/or thin plaques consisting of closely set or coalescing, skin-colored or brown, verrucous papules or pruritic, erythematous, and hyperkeratotic papules that often coalesce into plaques • Present at birth or develop in early childhood • Rarely reported to transform into basal cell and squamous cell carcinoma in adulthood
Nevus sebaceous (5)	• Congenital hamartoma of the skin • Waxy, yellow-orange or tan, well-circumscribed, hairless plaques that appear during infancy • Develops into deforming mass in adulthood • Potential for malignant transformation
Plexiform neurofibroma (6)	• Uncommon variant of neurofibromatosis type 1 • Plaquelike enlargement, usually on craniomaxillofacial region • Lesion texture: "bag of worms" • Other findings consistent with neurofibromatosis type 1
Urbach-Wiethe disease (lipoid proteinosis) (7)(8)	• Rare autosomal recessive genodermatosis • Characterized by persistent voice hoarseness in infancy and accompanied by skin changes (ie, fragility, discomfort, infiltrated papules, and/or nodules)

As new cases emerge, the criterion for diagnosis of NCM continues to be refined. Fox (15) was the first to recommend guidelines, and Kadonaga and Frieden (11) have recently suggested a revised definition, which requires the following 3 criteria to be met:

Criteria 1: having either 1 large or 3 or more CMN with associated meningeal melanosis or CNS melanoma with large defined as greater than or equal to 20 cm on an adult, greater than 9 cm on an infant scalp, or greater than or equal to 6 cm in diameter on an infant body.

Criteria 2: no evidence of cutaneous melanoma and meningeal lesions are histologically benign.

Criteria 3: no evidence of meningeal melanoma and cutaneous lesions are histologically benign. (11)

In asymptomatic patients at high-risk of NCM, those with large and/or giant CMN with satellite lesions or with multiple medium-sized CMN (≥2 lesions), it is recommended that infants be screened with a gadolinium-enhanced MRI of the brain and spine prior to 6 months of age. (16) This is especially important if the nevus overlies the posterior axis, as this puts them at highest risk for NCM. (14)(17)

NCM can be asymptomatic or present with multiple complications including, but not limited to, hydrocephalus, seizures, hypotonia, developmental delay, mass lesions, cord compression, and premature death. (11) Review of the literature reveals that when neurologic manifestations do occur in infants and children, they have a poor prognosis with rapid demise eventually leading to death. (18)(19) Unfortunately, there are no curative treatment options available at this time. However, palliative measures should be offered to these patients as early as possible.

Large and giant CMN also carry the potential for malignant transformation (cutaneous melanoma and extracutaneous melanoma); risk increases with nevus size. It is estimated that large and giant CMN carry a 2% to 40% lifetime risk of malignant transformation, and approximately one-half of these cases occur within the first 3 years of life. (20)(21) The highest risk is associated with CMN with a final size of greater than 40 cm and truncal location. (21) Furthermore, large and giant CMN have also been linked to a number of other malignancies including rhabdomyosarcoma, liposarcoma, and malignant peripheral sheath tumors. (22) Lastly, large and giant CMN are associated with negative psychosocial effects due to the appearance of such lesions. Therefore, patients' mental health should be monitored as they grow and appropriate resources offered. (23)

Patients and families often desire surgical removal of large and giant CMN due to risk of malignancy as well as cosmetic and psychosocial ramifications. Complete excision is not possible in many cases; however, resection can be beneficial for some. Factors that affect the decision for removal include the following: size, location, technical difficulty of the type of procedure required, and anesthesia options. (24) Even if complete removal is possible, it is important to note that this does not eliminate the risk of melanoma in the future as patients can develop melanoma within the CNS or retroperitoneum. (25)

PATIENT COURSE

The patient was discharged from the NICU and was seen in the pediatric out-patient clinic at 11 days of life for her first newborn visit. The patient's mother did not report any neurologic or dermatologic changes. The patient's head circumference remained stable and she gained weight appropriately. The patient is scheduled for a repeat MRI of the brain and to follow-up with neurology, dermatology, ophthalmology, and cardiology.

Summary

- CMN are common at birth. It is important for clinicians to recognize which CMN have increased risk for life-threatening consequences and warrant further evaluation.

- Large CMN in children are greater than 9 cm on the head or greater than 6 cm on the body and are expected to be 20 to 40 cm in adulthood. Giant CMN will grow to be greater than 40 cm in adults.

- Large and giant CMN are associated with NCM, malignant transformation, and negative psychosocial effects.

- Asymptomatic infants with a high-risk of NCM, those with large and/or giant CMN with satellite lesions or with 2 or more medium-sized CMN should be screened with a gadolinium-enhanced MRI of the brain and spine prior to 6 months of age (grade 2C).

- Surgical removal may be an option for some patients for both cosmetic and medical reasons. However, this does not remove the risk of neurological complications or malignancy in other organ systems.

References for this article can be found at https://doi.org/10.1542/pir.2018-0270.